**Pocket Guide
to Echocardiography**

Companion website

This book is accompanied by a companion website:

www.wiley.com/go/kacharava/echocardiography

The website includes:

- 64 Multiple-choice questions
- 68 Videos

Pocket Guide to Echocardiography

Andro G. Kacharava MD, PhD

Echocardiography Laboratory
Emory University School of Medicine
Atlanta VA Medical Center
Atlanta, GA, USA

Alexander T. Gedevanishvili, MD

Echocardiography Laboratory
Southern CardioPulmonary Associates
West Georgia Health System
LaGrange, GA, USA

Guram G. Imnadze, MD, PhD

Schuechtermann Klinik
Bad Rothenfelde, Germany

Dimitri M. Tsverava, MD

Tbilisi Medical Academy
MediClubGeorgia
Tbilisi, Georgia

Craig M. Brodsky, MD

Echocardiography Laboratory
Boca Raton Community Hospital
Boca Raton, FL, USA

FOREWORD BY

Navin C. Nanda

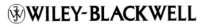

A John Wiley & Sons, Ltd., Publication

This edition first published 2012, © 2012 by John Wiley & Sons, Ltd.

Wiley-Blackwell is an imprint of John Wiley & Sons, formed by the merger of Wiley's global Scientific, Technical and Medical business with Blackwell Publishing.

Registered office: John Wiley & Sons, Ltd, The Atrium, Southern Gate, Chichester, West Sussex, PO19 8SQ, UK

Editorial offices: 9600 Garsington Road, Oxford, OX4 2DQ, UK
The Atrium, Southern Gate, Chichester, West Sussex, PO19 8SQ, UK
111 River Street, Hoboken, NJ 07030–5774, USA

For details of our global editorial offices, for customer services and for information about how to apply for permission to reuse the copyright material in this book please see our website at www.wiley.com/wiley-blackwell

ISBN: 9780470674444

A catalogue record for this book is available from the British Library.

Wiley also publishes its books in a variety of electronic formats. Some content that appears in print may not be available in electronic books.

Set in 7/9pt Frutiger Light by Thomson Digital, Noida, India
Printed in Singapore by Ho Printing Singapore Pte Ltd

1   2012

Contents

Foreword by Navin C. Nanda, vii
Preface, ix
Abbreviations, xi

1 Comprehensive transthoracic echocardiographic examination protocol, 1
2 Indications, contraindications and endpoints of dobutamine and exercise stress echocardiography, 6
3 Types of stress echocardiography and reading template, 8
4 Useful formulas and normal values, 10
5 Guidelines for the safe use of echocardiography contrast, 12
6 Atrial and ventricular dimensions, 13
7 Coronary artery disease, 21
8 Left ventricular systolic function and left ventricular diastolic patterns, 23
9 Right ventricular systolic function and right ventricular diastolic patterns, 27
10 Dilated, hypertrophic and restrictive cardiomyopathies, 30
11 Pericardial effusion, cardiac tamponade, constrictive pericarditis, 31
12 Mitral stenosis, 32
13 Mitral valvuloplasty score, 33
14 Recommendations for data recording and measurement for mitral stenosis, 34
15 Mitral regurgitation, 36
16 Aortic regurgitation, 38
17 Aortic stenosis, 39
18 Recommendations for data recording and measurement for aortic stenosis, 40
19 Resolution of apparent discrepancies in measures of aortic stenosis severity, 42
20 Pulmonic stenosis, pulmonic regurgitation, pulmonary hypertension, 43
21 Tricuspid regurgitation and tricuspid stenosis, 45
22 Infective endocarditis, 47
23 ACC/ASE recommendations for echocardiography in ineffective endocarditis, 48
24 Prosthetic valves, 49
25 Normal echocardiographic values for prosthetic valves, 51
26 Congenital heart disease, 53
27 Miscellaneous, 54
28 Aortic diseases, 55
29 Indication for surgery in aortic diseases, 56
30 Transthoracic echocardiographic and Doppler protocols for assessment of ventricular dyssynchrony, 57
31 Indications, contraindications and complications of transesophageal echocardiographic examination, 59
32 Routine approach to any transesophageal echocardiographic and recommended views for evaluation of aorta, 61

33 Terminology used to describe manipulation of the probe and transducer during image acquisition, 62

34 Diagrams of standard transesophageal echocardiographic views, 63

35 Transesophageal echocardiographic measurements, 64

36 Transesophageal echocardiographic diagram of the regional blood supply to cardiac wall segments, 67

37 Transesophageal echocardiographic orientation for assessment of the mitral valve, 68

38 Diagrams of transesophageal echocardiographic views in the evaluation of the mitral valve, 70

39 References and Recommended Literature, 72

Supplement to pocket guide of echocardiography, 75

A companion website with videos and MCQs is available at www.wiley.com/go/kacharava/echocardiography.

Companion website

This book is accompanied by a companion website:
www.wiley.com/go/kacharava/echocardiography

The website includes:
- 64 Multiple-choice questions
- 68 Video clips

Foreword

I am most pleased to write this Foreword for the book entitled "Pocket Guide of Echocardiography," first edition, authored by Andro Kacharava, Alexander Gedevanishvili, Guram Imnadze, Dimitri Tsverava, and Craig Brodsky. The book begins with a summary of the TTE examination protocol and a comprehensive listing of useful formulas and normal values. These are followed by atrial and ventricular dimensions, LV and RV systolic function, LV diastolic patterns and their usefulness in evaluating diastolic heart failure and echocardiographic findings in various types of cardiomyopathies, cardiac tamponade, and constrictive pericarditis. Valvular heart disease, pulmonary hypertension, infective endocarditis, prosthetic valves, congenital heart disease, and clinically useful aspects of transesophageal echocardiography are also covered. The book ends with a list of references useful to the reader. The book is supplemented by several excellent diagrams, illustrations and tables, as well as short video clips and self-assessment questions. This pocketbook book will prove a handy asset not only to students and medical residents but also practicing cardiologists and echocardiographers.

This is one of the best books of its type that I have seen and I would recommend it highly.

Navin C. Nanda, MD
Professor of Medicine and Director
Heart Station/Echocardiography Laboratories
University of Alabama at Birmingham, Birmingham, Alabama
President, International Society of Cardiovascular Ultrasound
Editor-in-Chief, *Echocardiography*: a journal of cardiovascular
ultrasound and allied techniques

Preface

More than half a century has passed since, on October 29, 1953, Inge Edler (a Swedish cardiologist) and Carl Helmut Hertz (a German physicist) recorded the first moving picture of the heart using a Siemens Ultrasound Reflectoscope, thus inaugurating the field of "ultrasound cardiography." Due to its easy accessibility, low cost, and fantastic ability to provide rapid quantitative information about the cardiac structure and function at the bedside, echocardiography has developed rapidly within the last 30 years. These qualities make it one of the major diagnostic tools in clinical cardiology.

This pocket guide does not attempt to provide a comprehensive review of echocardiography, as that is not its goal; instead we strongly recommended that young cardiologists should obtain detailed information on echocardiography topics from the many excellent major echocardiography textbooks available. The *Pocket Guide to Echocardiography* is primarily designed to provide a compact, yet practical, pocket guide addressing the key aspects in the field of everyday clinical cardiac ultrasound, and we hope that the condensed format will be particularly helpful during the routine daily interpretation of echocardiographic images. The pocket guide and its companion will help novice cardiologists to develop a stepwise approach in their interpretation of a standard transthoracic echocardiographic study, teach them how to, methodically, gather and assemble the important pieces of information from each of the standard echocardiographic views in order to generate a complete final report of the study performed. We also hope that the pocket guide will be of great assistance during busy night calls while performing emergent/urgent echocardiography studies.

In order to improve the visual comprehension of the echocardiographic images of different cardiac pathologies, a companion web site is included containing more than 60 video clips, each with a short description, demonstrating a wide range of cardiovascular pathology. In addition, the site also lists 68 multiple-choice questions, with subsequent correct answers, to help to consolidate the theoretical knowledge in the field of adult clinical echocardiography.

We would like to thank our teachers and colleagues for their support, encouragement, and work revising this manual. Many thanks to West Georgia Health cardiology department and the cardiology division of the Emory University School of Medicine. Our special thanks go to Dr. Navin C. Nanda who agreed to review our pocket guide and write a foreword to the book. We hope that the *Pocket Guide to Echocardiography* will be well recieved and prove useful to cardiac specialists, emergency medicine physicians, and anesthesiologists alike. We also hope that it will contribute to an improved standard of cardiac care for our patients.

Andro G. Kacharava
Alexander T. Gedevanishvili
Guram G. Imnadze
Dimitri M. Tsverava
Craig M. Brodsky

Abbreviations

A′	Annular diastolic A wave
A2C	Apical 2 Chambers
A4C	Apical 4 Chambers
AA	Aortic Area
AO	Aorta
AR	Aortic Regurgitation
ASD	Atrial Septal Defect
AT	Acceleration Time
AV	Aortic Valve also
AVA	Aortic Valve Area
AVRF	Aortic Valve Regurgitant Fraction
AVRV	Aortic Valve Regurgitant Volume
BSA	Body Surface Area
CABG	Coronary Artery Bypass Graft
CAD	Coronary Artery Disease
CO	Cardiac Output
CS	Coronary Sinus
CW	Continuous Wave
DBP	Diastolic Blood Pressure
DSE	Dobutamine Stress Echocardiography
DT	Deceleration Time
DTi	Doppler Tissue imaging
E′	Annular Diastolic E Wave
EF	Ejection Fraction
ERO	Effective Regurgitant Orifice
ESE	Exercise Stress Echocardiography
ET	Ejection Time
FS	Fractional Shortening
Hct	Hematocrit
Hgb	Hemoglobin
HR	Heart rate
HTN	Hypertension
HV	Hepatic Vein
IAS	Interatrial Septum
IVC	Inferior Vena Cava
IVRT	Isovolumic Ventricular Relaxation Time
IVS	Interventricular Septum
LA	Left Atrium
LAA	Left Atrial Appendage
LAD	Left Atrial Diameter
LAP	Left Atrial Pressure
LAX	Long Axis
LPA	Left Pulmonary Artery
LUPV	Left Upper Pulmonary Vein
LV dp/dt	Left Ventricular dp/dt

LV	Left Ventricle
LVEDD	Left Ventricular End Diastolic Diameter
LVEDP	Left Ventricular End Diastolic Pressure
LVESD	Left Ventricular End Systolic Diameter
LVOT	Left Ventricular Outflow Tract
LVPW	Left Ventricular Posterior Wall
MAC	Mitral Annular Calcification
ME	Mid Esophageal
MI	Myocardial Infarction
MPA	Main Pulmonary Artery
MR	Mitral Regurgitation
MS	Mitral Stenosis
MV	Mitral Valve
MVA	Mitral Valve Area
MVP	Mitral Valve Prolapse
MVRF	Mitral Valve Regurgitant Fraction
MVRV	Mitral Valve Regurgitant Volume
PA	Pulmonary Artery
PADP	Pulmonary Artery Diastolic Pressure
PAP	Pulmonary Artery Pressure
PAT	Pulmonary Acceleration Time
PBVP	Percutaneous Balloon Valvuloplasty
PCI	Percutaneous Coronary Intervention
PCWP	Pulmonary Capillary Wedge Pressure
PISA	Proximal Isovelocity Surface Area
PHT	Pressure Half Time
PR	Pulmonary Regurgitation
PR	Pulmonic Regurgitation
PS	Pulmonic Stenosis
PV	Pulmonic Valve
PVA	Pulmonary Vein Atrial Reversal Wave
PVR	Pulmonary Vascular Resistance
PVS1	Pulmonary Vein Systolic Wave 1
PVS2	Pulmonary Vein Systolic Wave 2
PW	Pulse Wave
RA	Right Atrium
RAP	Right Atrial Pressure
RPA	Right Pulmonary Artery
RUPV	Right Upper Pulmonary Vein
RV	Right Ventricle
RVOT	Right Ventricle Outflow
RVSP	Right Ventricular Systolic Pressure
RWT	Relative Wall Thickness
S′	Systolic Mitral Annular Velocity
SAM	Systolic Anterior Motion
SAX	Short Axis
SBP	Systolic Blood Pressure
SFR	Systolic Flow Reversal
Sn	Sensitivity

Sp	Specificity
SV	Stroke Volume
SVCc	Superior Vena Cava
SVT	Supraventricular Tachycardia
SWMA	Segmental Wall Motion Abnormalities
TAPSE	Tricuspid Annular Plane Systolic Excursion
TG	Trans Gastric
TR	Tricuspid Regurgitation
TRV	Tricuspid Regurgitation Velocity
TS	Tricuspid Stenosis
TV	Tricuspid Valve
TVA	Tricuspid Valve Area
UE	Upper Esophageal
Vp	Flow Propagation Velocity
VSD	Ventricular Septal Defect
VT	Ventricular Tachycardia
VTI	Velocity Time Integral
WMSI	Wall Motion Score Index

CHAPTER 1

Comprehensive transthoracic echocardiographic examination protocol

Parasternal long-axis view (Fig. 1)
1 2D image (4 beats) (measure LVOT diameter).
2 Color Doppler through MV and AoV (4 beats).
3 M-mode through Aortic root (measure root and LA diameter, and aortic cusp separation).
4 Color Doppler M-mode through the aortic root (4 beats).
5 M-mode through MV (± Valsalva test to check for MV prolapse and SAM; measure "E" to "S" separation distance).
6 Color Doppler M-mode through MV (4 beats).
7 M-mode through mid LV (4 beats) (measure septal and inferolateral wall thickness LVEDD and LVESD).

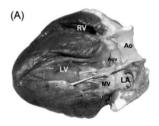 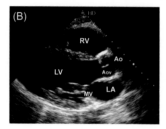

Figure 1 (A and B) Parasternal long-axis view.

RA/RV view
From parasternal LAX view tilt transducer to point it to right hip:
1 2D image (4 beats);
2 Color Doppler through TV (4 beats);
3 CW Doppler through TV to measure max TR velocity if TR jet present.

Parasternal short-axis view (Fig. 2 and Fig. 3)
1 2D through AoV (4 beats) (to assess structure and mobility; use zoom).
2 Color Doppler through AoV (4 beats).
3 2D through PV (4beats).
4 Color Doppler through PV (4 beats).
5 PW Doppler at the tips of PV to measure PAT (4 beats).

Pocket Guide to Echocardiography, First Edition. Andro G. Kacharava, Alexander T. Gedevanishvili, Guram G. Imnadze, Dimitri M. Tserava and Craig M. Brodsky.
© 2012 John Wiley & Sons, Ltd. Published 2012 by John Wiley & Sons, Ltd.

6 CW Doppler through PV to measure PR velocity if present, and maximum outflow velocity through PV.

7 2D through TV (4 beats).

8 Color Doppler through TV (4 beats).

9 PW Doppler at the tips of TV leaflets to assess inflow pattern (4 beats).

10 If inflow jet max velocity is >1.5 m/sec, trace the diastolic flow to measure mean transvalvular gradient.

11 CW Doppler through TV to measure max TR velocity if TR jet present.

12 Serial 2D short axis images through the LV from base toward apex.

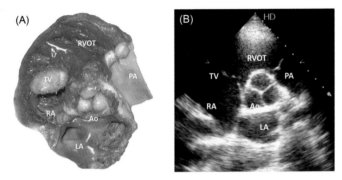

Figure 2 (A and B) Parasternal short-axis view.

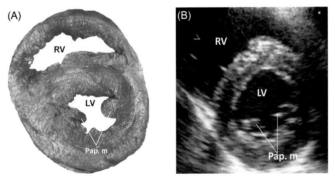

Figure 3 (A and B) Parasternal short-axis view.

Apical 4-chambers view (Fig. 4)

1 2D image (4 beats).
2 Color Doppler through the MV (4 beats).
3 Color Doppler M-mode through the MV at the end expiration (4 beats).
4 PW Doppler at the tips of MV leaflets to assess inflow pattern and velocity (4 beats); if pseudonormal or restrictive inflow pattern observed, decrease the preload and reassess the inflow pattern; in impaired relaxation act opposite.
5 PW Doppler at the right/left upper PV to assess inflow pattern (4 beats).
6 PW tissue Doppler at the basal and mid septal and lateral walls (4 beats).
7 If inflow jet max velocity is > 1.9 m/sec, trace the diastolic flow to measure mean transvalvular gradient, then measure PHT of the jet in CW mode.
8 CW Doppler through MV to measure max MR velocity if MR jet present. (Obtain simultaneous SBP measurement to calculate mean LAP.)
9 PW tissue Doppler at basal lateral walls of the RV to assess TEI index and systolic velocity.
10 M-mode through the RV basal lateral wall to measure TAPSE.

Apical 5-chambers view

From apical 4-chambers view tilt transducer slightly anteriorly; examiner's hand moves downward toward the patient's bed:

1 2D image (4 beats).
2 Color Doppler through AoV and MV (4 beats).
3 PW Doppler through LVOT and trace the flow (4 beats).
4 CW Doppler through AoV and if outflow max velocity is >1.9 m/sec, trace the flow for mean and peak gradients (4 beats).
5 CW Doppler through AoV to measure AR max velocity and pressure half-time if AR jet present. (Obtain simultaneous DBP measurement to calculate LV diastolic pressure.)

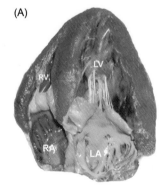
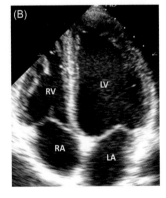

Figure 4 (A and B) Apical 4-chambers view.

Apical 2-chambers view (Fig. 5)

From apical 4-chambers view rotate transducer counter-clockwise until the RV is completely gone:

1 2D image (4 beats).

2 Color Doppler through the MV (4 beats).

3 PW tissue Doppler images at 4 points: basal and mid inferior, basal and mid anterior walls of the LV.

Apical 3-chambers view

From apical 2-chambers view rotate transducer counterclockwise and administer anterior tilt, examiner's hand moves downward toward the patient's bed, until the AoV comes into the view

1 2D image (4 beats).

2 Color Doppler through AoV and MV (4 beats).

3 PW Doppler through LVOT and trace the flow (4 beats).

4 CW Doppler through AoV and if outflow max velocity is >1.9 m/sec trace the flow for mean and peak gradients (4 beats).

5 CW Doppler through AoV to measure AI max velocity and pressure half-time if AI jet present. (Obtain simultaneous DBP measurement to calculate LV diastolic pressure.)

6 PW tissue Doppler images at 4 points: basal and mid anteroseptal, basal and mid inferolateral walls of the LV.

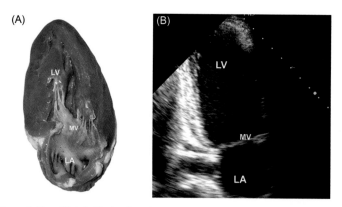

Figure 5 (A and B) Apical 2-chambers view.

Subcostal view

1 2D 4-chambers image with and without color Doppler over it (4 beats).

2 Color Doppler across the IAS and IVS.

3 Serial 2D short axis images through the LV from base toward apex.

4 PW Doppler of the hepatic vein.
5 Measure IVC diameter on inspiration and expiration.

Suprasternal notch view

1 2D image (4 beats).
2 PW and CW Doppler through discending and ascending Aorta.
3 Color Doppler through discending and ascending Aorta.

CHAPTER 2

Indications, contraindications and endpoints of dobutamine and exercise stress echocardiography

Indications for DSE/ESE

1 Evaluation of known or suspected CAD (a. Use tissue harmonic imaging; b. Intravenous contrast agent used if ≥ 2 myocardial segments are not well visualized).
2 Risk stratification prior to noncardiac surgery.
3 Risk stratification post MI, PCI, CABG.
4 Assessment of myocardial viability.
5 Evaluation of valvular hemodynamics.*
6 Evaluation of pulmonary hypertension.
7 Evaluation of unexplained dyspnea.

Contraindications

Absolute

1 MI<48 hours.
2 Unstable angina (chest pain <12 hours).
3 Absolute intolerance to dobutamine/beta-blockers/nitro.
4 Symptomatic arrhythmias.
5 Uncooperative or unwilling patient.
6 Active sepsis/endocarditis.
7 Severe metabolic/electrolyte abnormalities.
8 Highly mobile intracardiac mass.
9 Uncontrolled seizure disorder.
10 Known pregnancy.
11 Poor TTE images even with echocontrast.
12 Hemodynamic instability.
13 Hypertensive patient (SBP >200 mmHg, DBP >110 mmHg).
14 Inability to exercise (consider DSE).
15 Severe symptomatic valvular disease.

Relative

1 LVEF < 25%, except for viability studies.
2 Pulmonary HTN (mean PAP >50 mmHg, or peak PAP > 70 mmHg).
3 Hypertrophic obstructive cardiomyopathy.
4 Severe asymptomatic valvular disease.
5 Large aortic aneurysms.
6 Anemia (Hct <30, Hgb <10).

Endpoints

1 Achieved target heart rate.
2 Peak dobutamine injection rate according to the protocol reached.

Pocket Guide to Echocardiography, First Edition. Andro G. Kacharava, Alexander T. Gedevanishvili, Guram G. Imnadze, Dimitri M. Tserava and Craig M. Brodsky.
© 2012 John Wiley & Sons, Ltd. Published 2012 by John Wiley & Sons, Ltd.

3 Development of significant arrhythmias (high degree AV block or SVT/VT).

4 Development of the well-documented new SWMA.

5 Development of hemodynamic instability/intolerable symptoms.

6 Patient refusal to proceed further at any point of the test.

7 Hypotension.

*Stress echocardiography indicated in MV or AoV disease

1 Asymptomatic or minimally symptomatic patient with significant MV or AoV disease.

2 Disproportionally symptomatic patient in the absence of significant MV or AoV disease.

3 Assessment of myocardial reserve ($\uparrow$ in SV > 20%) with DSE in patients with low LVEF, and differentiation between true (eg. AVA < 1.0 cm^2 and mean AoV TVG < 30 mmHg) and pseudo-severe aortic stenosis.

Types of stress echo

1 Exercise stress echo:

  a Ischemia assessment.

  b Valvular disorder assessment.

  c Pulmonary HTN assessment.

  d Dynamic ventricular gradient assessment.

2 Dobutamine stress echo:

  a Ischemia assessment.

  b Myocardial viability assessment.

  c Valvular disorder assessment.

3 Vasodilator stress echo with hangrip exercise:

  a Ischemia assessment.

  b Myocardial viability assessment.

4 Pacing stress echo (transesophageal atrial pacing, or permanent pacemaker pacing $\pm$ Dobutamine):

  a Ischemia assessment.

  b Myocardial viability assessment.

CHAPTER 3

Types of stress echocardiography and reading template

Additional information
1 Type of exercise protocol and total exercise or medication infusion time.
2 Adequacy of stress echo (HR, BP, Double product).
3 Clinical symptoms at baseline, during and post stress echo.
4 Dose of pharmacologic agents used at the peak of the test.
5 Reason of termination of a study.
6 HR and BP at the time of occurance of SWMA.
7 Complications.

Baseline ECG description
1 Rhythm.
2 Rate.
3 Axis.
4 PR, QRS, QT length.
5 ST-T changes.

Stress ECG description
1 Rhythm.
2 Rate.
3 Axis.
4 PR, QRS, QT length.
5 ST-T changes.

Baseline echocardiography data description
1 LV cavity size and wall thickness.
2 RV cavity size and wall thickness.
3 Gross LV systolic function.
4 LVEF.
5 Gross RV systolic function.
6 LV SWM score.
7 RV wall motion.
8 RVSP.
9 LVOT peak gradient.
10 MV mean and peak gradient (in MS and prosthetic MV).
11 MR presence and severity.
12 AV area and mean gradient (in AS and prosthetic AoV).
13 Aortic Root and Ascending Aortic diameter.
14 LV Diastolic function:
  a E/E[1] ratio;
  b Mitral E wave DT.

Pocket Guide to Echocardiography, First Edition. Andro G. Kacharava, Alexander T. Gedevanishvili, Guram G. Imnadze, Dimitri M. Tsverava and Craig M. Brodsky.

Stress echocardiography data description

1 LV cavity size and wall thickness.
2 RV cavity size and wall thickness.
3 Gross LV systolic function.
4 LVEF.
5 Gross RV systolic function.
6 LV SWM score.
7 RV wall motion.
8 RVSP.
9 LVOT peak gradient.
10 MV mean and peak gradient (in MS and prosthetic MV).
11 MR presence and severity.
12 AV area and mean gradient (in AS and prosthetic AoV).
13 LV Diastolic function:
   a E/E^1 ratio;
   b Mitral E wave DT.

Final conclusion

1 Ischemia.
2 Viability.
3 Valvular disorder.
4 Pulmonary HTN.
5 Dynamic ventricular outflow gradient.

CHAPTER 4

Useful formulas and normal values

Useful formulas

LVEDP $= $ DBP $- 4V^2$, where V is max velocity of AI jet
LAP $= $ SBP $- 4V^2$, where V is max velocity of MR jet
LAP $= $ RAP $+ 4V^2$, where V is max velocity of ASD jet
SV $= $ Area$_{LVOT}$ $\times$ VTI$_{LVOT}$
CO $= $ HR $\times$ SV
PASP $= $ SBP $- 4V^2$, where V is velocity of PDA jet
PADP $= $ RAP $+ 4V^2$, where V is maximal end diastolic PI velocity
RVSP $= $ SBP $- 4V^2$, where V is velocity of VSD jet
RVSP $= $ RAP $+ 4V^2$, where V is max velocity of TR jet

Pericardial fluid volume (ml) $= P^3 - H^3$, where P is diameter of pericardial space in circumferential pericardial effusion, H is diameter of the heart in diastole (measurements in parasternal LAX view).
   Area of the MV annulus $= 0.785 \times$ D1 $\times$ D2, where D1 is diameter in 4-chambers view, and D2 in 2-chambers view.

$E/E^1 > 15 \rightarrow$ LVEDP > 19 mmHg (for medial mitral annulus)
$E/E^1 > 12 \rightarrow$ LVEDP > 19 mmHg (for lateral mitral annulus)
If LVEF $<50\%$, E/A >2, DT <160 msec $\rightarrow$ PCWP >18 mmHg
PCWP $= 5.27 \times$ E/Vp $+ 4.6$
PCWP $= 1.55 + 1.47 \times E/E^1$ (sinus tachycardia)
PCWP $= 1.9 + 1.24 \times E/E^1$ (normal sinus rhythm)

If E/Vp $> 2.5 \rightarrow$ PCWP > 15 mmHg, where Vp is a mitral inflow propagation velocity in color M-mode, E is MV inflow E wave velocity, and E^1 is MV annulus early diastolic velocity (all measurements done at end expiration)

PAP$_{mean}$ $= [79 - (0.45 \times$ PAT$)]$ (use only if HR 60-90)
PAP$_{mean}$ $= 0.65 \times$ PASP $+ 0.55$
PVR $= $ TR velocity (m/sec)/TVIRVOT (cm) $\times 10 + 0.16$ (Woods units)
LVEF $= 1.7 \times$ FS, in the absence of SWMA

LVEF $= 2.8 \times$ LVOT TVI, in the absence of severe diastolic dysfunction, significant VSD, MR, AI, dilated or very small LV cavity

Pocket Guide to Echocardiography, First Edition. Andro G. Kacharava, Alexander T. Gedevanishvili, Guram G. Imnadze, Dimitri M. Tsverava and Craig M. Brodsky.
© 2012 John Wiley & Sons, Ltd. Published 2012 by John Wiley & Sons, Ltd.

LVEF	dP/dt
Normal	> 1200 mmHg/s
Mildly depressed	1000–1200 mmHg/s
Moderately depressed	800–999 mmHg/s
Severely depressed	< 800 mmHg/s

RVEF	dP/dt
Normal	> 400 mmHg/s

Normal values

Aorta at:	
Sinuses of Valsalva	2.1–3.5 cm
Sinotubular junction	1.7–3.4 cm
Ascending segment	2.1–3.5 cm; wall thickness ≤ 3.0 mm
Descending segment	1.4–3.0 cm; wall thickness ≤ 5.0 mm
Peak aortic flow velocity	71–120 cm/s
LVEF	≥ 55%
LVOT	1.4–2.6 cm
RVOT (above AoV)	2.5–2.9 cm; (above PV): 1.7–2.3
MPA (below PV)	1.5–2.1 cm
RPA	0.9–1.3 cm
LPA	0.8–1.6 cm
CS	0.4–1.0 cm
LA	2.3–3.9 cm
RA	2.5–4.1 cm
Peak E velocity	0.60–0.68 m/s
Peak A velocity	0.38–0.48 m/s
E/A ratio	1.5–2.0
LVEDD	3.6–5.5 cm
LVESD	2.3–3.8 cm
RV thickness	≤ 0.6 cm
Posterior LV wall thickness	0.6–1.0 cm
IVS thickness	0.6–1.0 cm
E/E[1]	< 8

CHAPTER 5

Guidelines for the safe use
of echocardiography contrast

Patients with pulmonary hypertension or unstable cardiopulmonary conditions should be monitored with vital sign measurements, electrocardiography and cutaneous oxygen saturation during and at least 30 minutes after administration of the products. All other patients should be observed closely during and after administration of the products.

Resuscitation equipment and trained personnel should always be readily available during the drug administration and monitoring period.

Contraindications

DefinityR® is contraindicated among patients with either known hypersensitivity to the products (Optison® is contraindicated among patients with known hypersensitivity to blood products and albumin) or have fixed right-to-left, bi-directional cardiac shunts or transient right-to-left shunts. Definity® should not be given intra-arterially.

Clinical applications

1 Precise quantification of LV volumes, LVEF, LV SWMA at baseline and with stress.
2 Accurate definition of cardiac anatomy:apical hypertrophy, noncompaction, thrombus, Tako-Tsubo, LV aneurysm and pseudoaneurysm, myocardial rupture, intracardiac mass.
3 Doppler enhancement.
4 Alcohol septal ablation.

Pocket Guide to Echocardiography, First Edition. Andro G. Kacharava, Alexander T. Gedevanishvili, Guram G. Imnadze, Dimitri M. Tsverava and Craig M. Brodsky.
© 2012 John Wiley & Sons, Ltd. Published 2012 by John Wiley & Sons, Ltd.

CHAPTER 6
Atrial and ventricular dimensions

LV Hypertrophy

	Mild	Moderate	Severe
IVSd (cm)	1.1–1.3	1.4–1.6	≥1.7
LVPWd (cm)	1.1–1.3	1.4–1.6	≥1.7
LV mass/BSA (g/m²)	116–131	132–148	≥149

Relative Wall Thickness (RWT) = 2 × LVPWd/LVIDd,

In the presence of increased LV mass	RWT ≥ 0.42 suggests concentric LVH
	RWT < 0.42 suggests eccentric LVH

LV dilatation:	Mild	Moderate	Severe
LVEDD (cm)	5.6–6.2	6.3–6.9	≥7.0

LV volume index (ml/m²):	Mild	Moderate	Severe
LV diastolic volume/BSA	76–86	87–96	≥97
LV systolic volume/BSA	31–36	37–42	≥43

RV Dilatation
- RV sharing the apex in the 4-chambers view.
- RV larger than LV in the subcostal view.
- RV nearly equal or larger than LV in the precordial views.
- RV size ≥ the 2/3 LV size in 4-chambers view – RV mildly dilated.
- RV size = the LV size in 4-chambers view – RV moderately dilated.
- RV size > than LV size in 4-chambers view – RV severely dilated.

Pocket Guide to Echocardiography, First Edition. Andro G. Kacharava, Alexander T. Gedevanishvili, Guram G. Imnadze, Dimitri M. Tsverava and Craig M. Brodsky.

LA Volume Index (LA volume/BSA)

Normal	16–28 ml/m^2
Mild dilatation	29–33 ml/m^2
Moderate dilatation	34–39 ml/m^2
Severe dilatation	>40 ml/m^2

LA volume = $\pi/6 \times L \times D1 \times D2$ (diameter method)
LA volume = $0.85 \times A^1 \times A^2/L$ (area method)

where:
D1 and D2 are diameters of the LA in parasternal long and short views.
A^1 is LA area in 4-chambers view.
A^2 is LA area in 2-chambers view.
L represents length of LA in 4-chambers view.[*]
[*] The L in 2-chambers view should not differ by >20%.

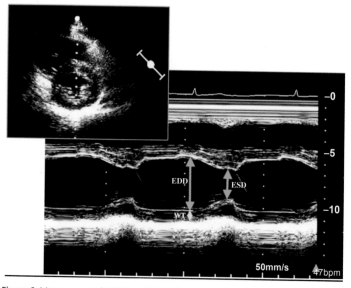

Figure 6 Measurement of LVEDD and LVESD from M-mode, Guided by parasternal short-axis image (upper left). (Reproduced, with permission, from Lang et al., 2005.)

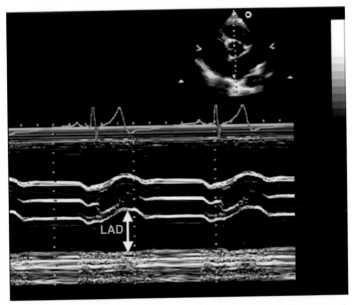

Figure 7 Measurement of left atrial diameter (LAD) from M-mode, Guided by parasternal short-axis image (upper right) at level of aortic valve. (Reproduced, with permission, from Lang et al., 2005.)

	Dilatation			
	Normal	**Mild**	**Moderate**	**Severe**
RVD1 (cm)	2.0–2.8	2.9–3.3	3.4–3.8	≥3.9
RVD2 (cm)	2.7–3.3	3.4–3.7	3.8–4.1	≥4.2
RVD3 (cm)	7.1–7.9	8.0–8.5	8.6–9.1	≥9.2
RVDA (cm^2)	11–28	29–32	33–37	≥38
RVSA (cm^2)	7.5–16	17–19	20–22	≥23
RVOT1 (cm)	2.5–2.9	3.0–3.2	3.3–3.5	≥3.6
RVOT2 (cm)	1.7–2.3	2.4–2.7	2.8–3.1	≥3.2
PA1 (cm)	1.5–2.1	2.2–2.5	2.6–2.9	≥3.0

RV Fractional area change (%):	Normal:	32–60
	Mildly depressed:	25–31
	Moderately depressed:	18–24
	Severely depressed:	≤17

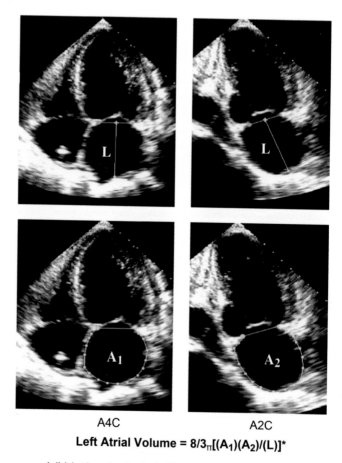

A4C   A2C

Left Atrial Volume = $8/3_\pi[(A_1)(A_2)/(L)]$*

* (L) is the shortest of either the A4C or A2C length

Figure 8 Measurement of left atrial (LA) Volume from area-length (L) method using apical 4-chambers (A4C) and apical 2-chambers (A2C) views at ventricular end systole (maximum LA size). L is measured from back wall to line across hinge points of mitral valve. Shorter L from either A4C or A2C is used in equation. (Reproduced, with permission, from Lang et al., 2005.)

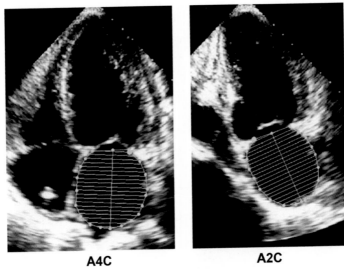

A4C   **A2C**

Figure 9 Measurement of left atrial (LA) volume from biplane method of disks (modified Simpson's Rule) Using apical 4-chambers (A4C) and apical 2-chambers (A2C) views at ventricular end systole (maximum LA size). (Reproduced, with permission, from Lang et al., 2005.)

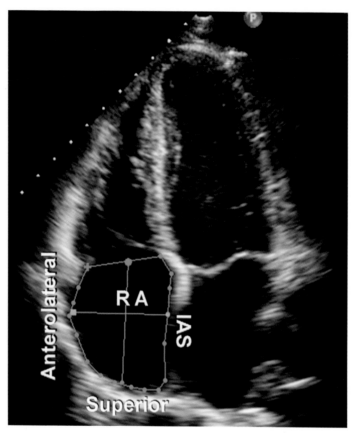

Figure 10 Measurement of right atrial (RA) diameters and area using apical 4-chambers (A4C) views at ventricular end systole (maximum RA size). RA major dimension < 5.4 cm (normal); RA minor dimension < 4.5 cm (normal); RA end-systolic area ≤ 18 cm² (normal). (Reproduced, with permission, from Rudski et al., 2010.)

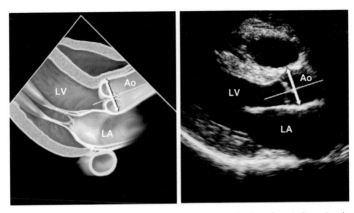

Figure 11 Measurement of aortic root diameter at sinuses of valsava from 2-dimensional parasternal long-axis image. Although leading edge to leading edge technique is shown, some prefer inner edge to inner edge method. (Reproduced, with permission, from Lang et al., 2005.)

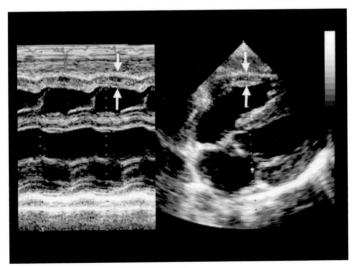

Figure 12 Methods of measuring right ventricular wall thickness (arrows) from M-mode (left) and subcostal transthoracic (right) echocardiograms. (Reproduced, with permission, from Lang et al., 2005.)

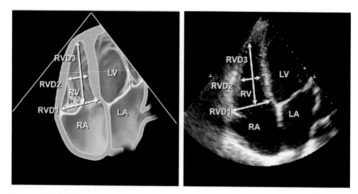

Figure 13 Mid right ventricular diameter measured in apical 4-chambers view at level of left ventricular papillary muscles. (Reproduced, with permission, from Lang et al., 2005.)

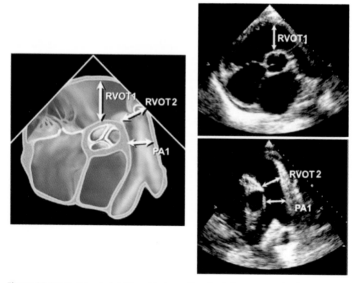

Figure 14 Measurement of right ventricular outflow tract diameter at subpulmonary region (RVOT1) and pulmonic valve annulus (RVOT2) in aortic valve short-axis view. (Reproduced, with permission, from Lang et al., 2005.)

CHAPTER 7

Coronary artery disease

Wall motion score (WMSI): (sum of scores/no. of segments visualized).
Normal 0, mild 1, moderate 2, severe 3, dyskinesis 4, aneurysm 5.
WMSI > 1.7 suggests that > 20% of myocardium is damaged or under the risk.
Old MI (scar): thinned, akinetic, dense tissue.
Acute MI: normal diastolic thickness, but absence of systolic thickening.

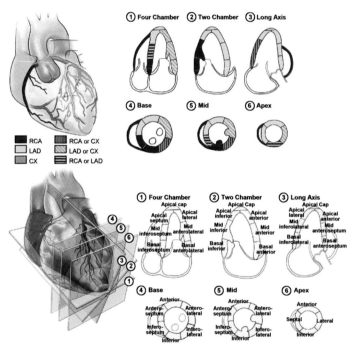

Figure 15 Typical distributions of coronary arteries with segmental analysis of LV walls based on schematic views, in parasternal short- and long-axis orientation, at 3 different levels. (Reproduced, with permission, from Lang et al., 2005.)

Pocket Guide to Echocardiography, First Edition. Andro G. Kacharava, Alexander T. Gedevanishvili, Guram G. Imnadze, Dimitri M. Tsverava and Craig M. Brodsky.
© 2012 John Wiley & Sons, Ltd. Published 2012 by John Wiley & Sons, Ltd.

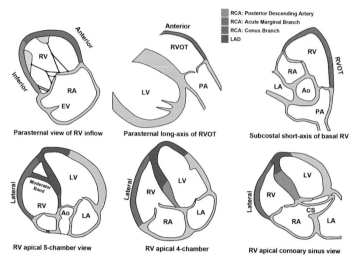

Figure 16 Segmental nomenclature of RV walls, along with their coronary supply. (Reproduced, with permission, from Rudski et al., 2010.)

CHAPTER 8
Left ventricular systolic function and left ventricular diastolic patterns

Left ventricular systolic function

	Normal
LV dP/dT	$\geq$ 1200 mmHg/sec
Fractional Shortening	$\geq$ 30%
VTI of LVOT	18–22
VTI of MV	10–13

$S^1 < 3.0$ cm/sec and $E^1 < 3.0$ cm/sec – high cardiac mortality predictors

$S^1 > 7.5$ cm/sec (peak myocardial systolic velocity averaged from 6 points around mitral valve annulus) – suggests grossly normal LVEF

M-mode markers of decreased LV systolic function:
- E-Septal separation > 2.5 cm implies EF < 25%;
- Closure drift of the AV at the end systole;
- Flattening of the posterior aorta;
- E-Septal separation > 0.6 cm suggests decreased EF.

Left ventricular diastolic patterns
- Mitral inflow assessed 20° lateral to apex, between the tips of leaflets.
- Pulmonary vein flow assessed 1.5 cm into the RUPV.
- Hepatic vein flow assessed 1–2 cm prox to junction with IVC.
- DT: deceleration time, extrapolated from peak of "E" wave to baseline.
- IVRT: isovolumetric relaxation time (from AV closure to MV opening; parallels DT).
- mA/pa: relative duration of mitral "A" wave to PV "a" wave;
  pVs1: atrial relaxation;
  pVs2: late flow into the LA in vent systole; (pVs1 & pVs2 are fused in 70%);
  pVd: mitral opening (mirrors "E" wave of MV flow, ↓DTof pVd with ↑ LVEDP);
  pVa: atrial systole → flow reversal (peak & duration ↑ with ↑ LVEDP).
- Hepatic, and SVC flow velocities: "S" (syst forward flow), "SR" (syst flow reversal), "D" (diastolic flow), "DR" (diast flow reversal).

Pocket Guide to Echocardiography, First Edition. Andro G. Kacharava, Alexander T. Gedevanishvili, Guram G. Imnadze, Dimitri M. Tsverava and Craig M. Brodsky.
© 2012 John Wiley & Sons, Ltd. Published 2012 by John Wiley & Sons, Ltd.

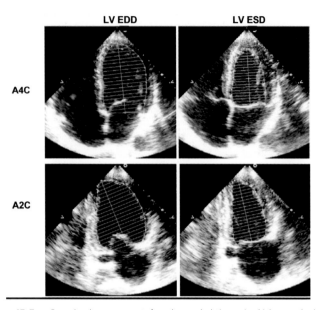

Figure 17 Two-dimensional measurements for volume calculations using biplane method of disks (modified Simpson's Rule) in apical 4-chambers (A4C) and apical 2-chambers (A2C) views at end diastole (LV EDD) and at end systole (LV ESD). Papillary muscles should be excluded from the cavity in the tracing. (Reproduced, with permission, from Lang et al., 2005.)

	E/A	DT (msc)	IVRT (msc)	mA/pVa pVa (m/s)	pV flow	
1 Normal:	>1	>160	70–90	>1	<0.25	≤1 pV D/pVS
2 Impaired relaxation:	<1	>240	>90	varies	<0.25	↑ DTof pVd, ↑ A
3 Pseudonormalization:	>1	>160	>60	<1	>0.25	↓DTof pVd, ↑pVa
4 Restrictive filling:	≥2	<160	<70	<1	>0.25	pVd ≫ pVs2
5 Constriction:	chgs c resp	<160	<70	<1	>0.25	chgs c resp

Tissue PW Doppler (basal septal and lateral walls)

$E^1/A^1 < 1 \rightarrow$ Diastolic dysfunction.

$E^1 =$ early diastolic mitral annulus velocity by tissue Doppler.

$A^1 =$ late diastolic mitral annulus velocity by tissue Doppler.

	E¹ velocity (septal annulus)	E¹ velocity (lateral annulus)
Restrictive	< 8 cm/s	< 10 cm/s
Normal/grey zone	8–11 cm/s	10–12 cm/s
Constrictive	≥ 12 cm/s	> 12 cm/s

Color M-mode (mitral inflow)

Vp > 50 cm/s → Normal, Vp is color M-mode Doppler mitral inflow propagation velocity.
Vp < 50 cm/s → Restrictive for young person; Vp < 40 cm/s for old person.
Vp > 100 cm/s → Constrictive.

Pressure	IVC	IVC change c respiration
0–5	< 1.5	Collapse
6–10	1.5–2.5	Decrease > 50%
11–15	1.5–2.5	Decrease < 50%
16–20	> 2.5	Decrease < 50%
> 20	> 2.5	No change

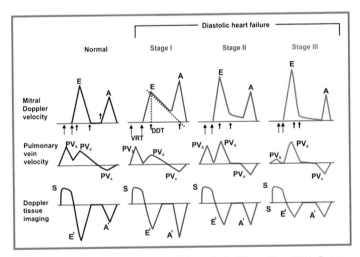

Figure 18 Echocardiographic assessment of left ventricular filling pattern. VRT indicates isovolumic relaxation time; DD T indicates E-wave deceleration time; E, early mitral inflow filling velocity; A, late mitral inflow velocity by atrial contraction; PVs, systolic pulmonary vein velocity; PVd, diastolic pulmonary vein velocity; PVa, pulmonary vein velocity from atrial contraction; S, myocardial velocity during systole; E′, myocardial velocity during early filling; A′, myocardial velocity during filling due to atrial contraction.

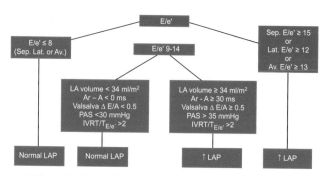

Figure 19 Diagnostic algorithm for the estimation of LV filling pressures in patients with normal LVEF. (Reproduced, with permission, from Nagueh et al., 2009.)

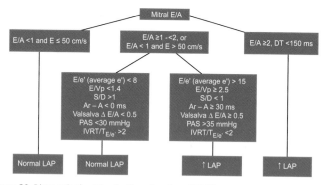

Figure 20 Diagnostic algorithm for the estimation of LV filling pressures in patients with depressed LVEF. (Reproduced, with permission, from Nagueh et al., 2009.)

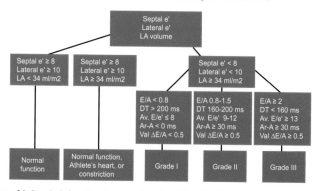

Figure 21 Practical algorithm to grade diastolic dysfunction. (Reproduced, with permission, from Nagueh et al., 2009.)

CHAPTER 9

Right ventricular systolic function and right ventricular diastolic patterns

Right ventricular diastolic patterns
Abnormal
If E/A ratio — <1.0 and E'/A' < 1.0, mild (Stage I) diastolic dysfunction is present.
E/E[1] ratio — > 6.0 & deceleration time (ms) < 120 suggest elevation of RV filling pressures.
If E/A ratio — <1.0 & S < D on hepatic flow, moderate (Stage II) diastolic dysfunction is present.
If E/A ratio — <1.0 & ↑ S reversal on hepatic flow in the absence of severe TR, severe (Stage III) diastolic dysfunction is present.

Right ventricular systolic function
1 TDI at the level of the TV annulus of the RV free wall – value of <10 cm/s identifies the presence of RV dysfunction with a Sn of 90% and Sp of 85%.
2 Tricuspid annular plane systolic excursion (TAPSE) – measures level of systolic excursion of the lateral TV annulus towards the apex in the 4 chambers view (measured with M-mode from apex to TV annulus at the RV free wall). In general, TAPSE < 1.6 cm is associated with decreased RV function, while ≥ 2.0 cm suggests normal function.
3 Myocardial Performance index = TCO – ET/ET = ICT + IRT/ET, if > 0.40, suggests ↓ RVEF.

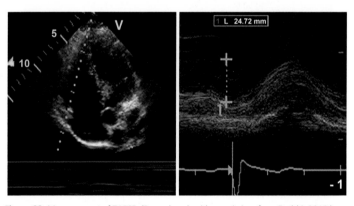

Figure 22 Measurement of TAPSE. (Reproduced, with permission, from Rudski, 2010.)

Pocket Guide to Echocardiography, First Edition. Andro G. Kacharava, Alexander T. Gedevanishvili, Guram G. Imnadze, Dimitri M. Tsverava and Craig M. Brodsky.
© 2012 John Wiley & Sons, Ltd. Published 2012 by John Wiley & Sons, Ltd.

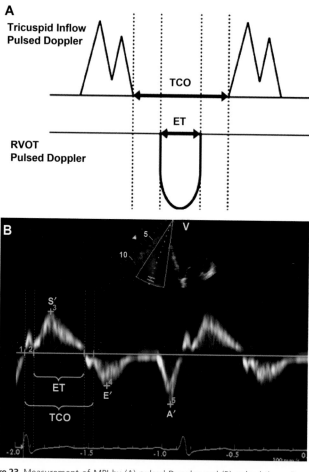

Figure 23 Measurement of MPI by (A) pulsed Doppler and (B) pulsed tissue Doppler. Tissue MPI, if > 0.5, suggests ↓ RVEF. (Reproduced, with permission, from Rudski, 2010.)

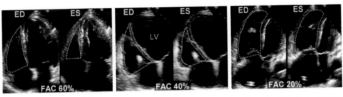

Figure 24 Measurement of FAC. (Reproduced, with permission, from Rudski et al., 2010.)

4 Fractional area change (FAC) <35% is abnormal.

Percentage FAC = 100% × {[end-diastolic area (Area ED) − end-systolic area (Area ES)]/end-diastolic area}

The endocardial border traced in apical 4-chambers (A4C) views from the tricuspid annulus along the free wall to the apex, then back to the annulus, along the interventricular septum at end-diastole (ED) and end-systole (ES). Trabeculation, tricuspid leaflets, and chords are included in the chamber: (left) normal subject, FAC 60%; (middle) moderately dilated right ventricle (RV), FAC 40%; (right) severely dilated RV, FAC 20%.

Dilated, hypertrophic and restrictive cardiomyopathies

Dilated cardiomyopathy
- LV/RV size increased, global hypokinesis (SWMA may present), mural thrombus.
- Low CO causes decreased MV separation, AV cusp closure is tapered.
- Spontaneous echo contrast in LV on 2D images.
- Diastole: impaired relaxation;pseudonormal or restrictive pattern if more advanced.

Hypertrophic cardiomyopathy
Myocardium appears granular; cavity is small, with near complete systolic obliteration.
- **SAM**: systolic anterior motion of mitral valve (ejection of blood creates a Bernoulli effect, shifting in the MV anterior leaflet, creating the dynamic LVOT obstruction; obstruction localized with PW Doppler; Doppler color aliasing occurs at the site as well).
- **Late systolic MR**: may be severe, usually posteriorly directed eccentric jet.
- Severity of obstruction is assessed with CW; delayed peak with "dagger"-shaped envelop; identify the isovolumic relaxation period to verify that the flow envelop is from the outflow tract, rather than MR jet.
- Gradient increased by Valsalva maneuver and in post PVC beat.
- Diastolic dysfunction occurs; impaired relaxation more common than restrictive pattern.

Restrictive cardiomyopathy
- Ventricular systolic fxn and size are normal, biatrial enlargement, MR, TR often present.
- Restrictive pattern on diastolic testing (E $\gg$ A, DT < 160 ms, IVRT < 60 ms).
- E^1 velocity < 8 cm/s on tissue Doppler.
- Vp < 50 cm/s (Vp is color M-mode Doppler flow propagation velocity through the mitral valve) → Restrictive for young person; Vp < 40 cm/s for old person.
- Restrictive diastolic pattern, occasionally diastolic mitral and tricuspid regurgitation occur.

Pocket Guide to Echocardiography, First Edition. Andro G. Kacharava, Alexander T. Gedevanishvili, Guram G. Imnadze, Dimitri M. Tsverava and Craig M. Brodsky.
© 2012 John Wiley & Sons, Ltd. Published 2012 by John Wiley & Sons, Ltd.

CHAPTER 11

Pericardial effusion, cardiac tamponade, constrictive pericarditis

Pericardial effusion

Small posterior, < 1 cm;
Medium circumferential, < 1.5 cm;
Large circumferential, ≥ 1.5 cm;
Epicardial fat small, anterior echo free space, absence of posterior echo free space;
Pericardial fluid excludes aorta; Pleural fluid wraps around it.

Cardiac tamponade

- RV early diastolic collapse; RA late diastolic and early systolic collapse;
- Inspiration decreases PVen, MV forward flow, LA, LV size; opposite c expiration;
- Inspiration increases HV, TV forward flow, RA, RV size; opposite c expiration and increase of flow reversal;
- LV IVRT (isovolumetric relaxation time) increases c inspiration; opposite c expiration;
- IVC engorged > 2 cm, non-pulsatile, no change c inspiration.

Constrictive pericarditis

- Pericardium bright, thickened ≥ 4 mm;
- Atria not markedly enlarged;
- Vp > 100 cm/sec (Vp is color M-mode Doppler flow propagation velocity through the Mitral valve);
- E^1 velocity > 8 cm/sec on tissue Doppler;
- LV IVRT (isovolumetric relaxation time) increases c inspiration; opposite c expiration;
- DT (deceleration time) of TV forward flow increases with inspiration; opposite with expiration;
- "Ventricular interdependence" inspiration => MV flow decreases => LV decreases => Septum shifts to the left => RV enlarges; opposite c expiration;
  Inspiration decreases PVen, MV flows, LA, LV size; opposite c expiration;
  Inspiration increases TV, PV flows, RA, RV size; opposite c expiration
  Expiration increases hepatic vein systolic and diastolic reversal flow
- IVC engorged > 2 cm, non-pulsatile, no change c inspiration.

Pocket Guide to Echocardiography, First Edition. Andro G. Kacharava, Alexander T. Gedevanishvili, Guram G. Imnadze, Dimitri M. Tsverava and Craig M. Brodsky.
© 2012 John Wiley & Sons, Ltd. Published 2012 by John Wiley & Sons, Ltd.

CHAPTER 12

Mitral stenosis

- MV morphology (valvular & subvalvular thickening, calcification, leaflet mobility).

Features of **rheumatic mitral stenosis**:
- Thickened calcified valve;
- "Hockey stick" appearance of anterior leaflet;
- Posterior leaflet immobile or tethered to anterior leaflet;
- "Fish mouth" orifice on parasternal SAX view;
- Decreased E-F slope on M-mode.

Gradient
- Max velocity (PW; CW; if aliases, use color to guide);
- Max gradient (by modified Bernoulli eq. $4V^2$);
- Mean gradient (by TVI in CW);
  Spontaneous contrast in LA in the absence of A.fib → at least moderate MS;
  Increase of MVmean TVG > 15 mmHg and/or RVSP > 60 mmHg during ESE suggests clinically significant MS.

Area
- Planimetry in parasternal SAX at the level of tips of the MV leaflets method;
- Continuity equation method (must use TVI b/c MV and LVOT ejection periods differ; cannot use if significant AI and/or MR exist);
- Pressure half time method (MVA = 220/PHT); MVA = 759/DT; (cannot use those formulas in: prosthetic valves with orifice areas > 1.5 cm²; presence of severe acute AI; and immediately s/p PBVP);
- Proximal isovelocity surface area (PISA) method;

- $$MVA = 2\pi r^2 * \frac{V_r}{V_{Max}} * \frac{\alpha^0}{180^0}$$

  $2\pi r^2$ Proximal isovelocity hemispheric surface area at a radial distance "r" from the MV orifice;
  V_r   Aliasing velocity at the radial distance "r" [cm/s];
  V_{Max}   Peak mitral stenosis velocity by CW [m/s];
  α   Angle between two mitral leaflets on the atrial side [degree];
  MVA   Mitral valve area [cm²].

Severity of MS

	MV area	Mean gradient	PHT
Normal	4.0–6.0 cm²	–	–
Mild	1.5–2.0 cm²	<5 mmHg	<150 ms
Moderate	1.0–1.5 cm²	5–10 mmHg	150–220 ms
Severe	<1.0 cm²	>10 mmHg	>220 ms

Pocket Guide to Echocardiography, First Edition. Andro G. Kacharava, Alexander T. Gedevanishvili, Guram G. Imnadze, Dimitri M. Tsverava and Craig M. Brodsky.
© 2012 John Wiley & Sons, Ltd. Published 2012 by John Wiley & Sons, Ltd.

CHAPTER 13
Mitral valvuloplasty score

Mitral valve score = Leaflet mobility + Valve thickening + Calcification + Subvalvular thickening

Item	Rating	Value Reduced mobility
Leaflet mobility	Highly mobile	1
	Basal leaflet motion only	3
	Minimal motion	4
Valve thickening	Near normal (4–5 mm)	1
	Thickened tips	2
	Entire leaflet thickened (5–8 mm)	3
	Marked leaflet thickening (>8–10 mm)	4
Calcification	Single area of brightness	1
	Scattered areas at leaflet margins	2
	Brightness extends to mid leaflets	3
	Extensive leaflet brightness	4
Subvalvular thickening	Minimal chordal thickening	1
	Chordal thickening up to 1/3	2
	Distal third of chordae thickening	3
	Extensive thickening to pap muscle	4
Mitral valve score	[No unit]	
Outcome	A score greater or equal to 8 is deemed "Poor".	
	A score lower than 8 is deemed "Good"	

Following parameters suggest ↑ mean LAP in patients with MS:
1 IVRT (< 60 ms has high specificity)
2 IVRT/TE-E' (< 4.2);
3 Mitral "A" wave velocity (>1.5 m/s).

Pocket Guide to Echocardiography, First Edition. Andro G. Kacharava, Alexander T. Gedevanishvili, Guram G. Imnadze, Dimitri M. Tsverava and Craig M. Brodsky.
© 2012 John Wiley & Sons, Ltd. Published 2012 by John Wiley & Sons, Ltd.

Recommendations for data recording and measurement for mitral stenosis

Data element	Recording	Measurement
Planimetry	• 2D parasternal short-axis view	• Contour of the inner mitral orifice
	• Determine the smallest orifice by scanning from apex to base	• Include commissures when opened
	• Positioning of measurement plan can be oriented by 3D echo	• In mid-diastole (use cine-loop)
	• Lowest gain setting to visualize the whole mitral orifice	• Average measurements if atrial fibrillation
Mitral flow	• Continuous-wave Doppler	• Mean gradient from the traced contour of the diastolic mitral flow
	• Apical windows often suitable (optimize intercept angle)	• Pressure half-time from the descending slope of the E-wave (mid-diastole slope if not linear)
	• Adjust gain setting to obtain well-defined flow contour	• Average measurements if atrial fibrillation
Systolic pulmonary artery pressure	• Continuous-wave Doppler	• Maximum velocity of tricuspid regurgitant flow
	• Multiple acoustic windows to optimize intercept angle	• Estimation of right atrial pressure according to inferior vena cava diameter
Valve anatomy	• Parasternal short-axis view	• Valve thickness (maximum and heterogeneity)
		• Commissural fusion
		• Extension and location of localized bright zones (fibrous nodules or calcification)
	• Parasternal long-axis view	• Valve thickness
		• Extension of calcification
		• Valve pliability
		• Subvalvular apparatus (chordal thickening, fusion, or shortening)
	• Apical two-chamber view	• Subvalvular apparatus (chordal thickening, fusion, or shortening)
		Detail each component and summarize in a score

Pocket Guide to Echocardiography, First Edition. Andro G. Kacharava, Alexander T. Gedevanishvili, Guram G. Imnadze, Dimitri M. Tsverava and Craig M. Brodsky.
© 2012 John Wiley & Sons, Ltd. Published 2012 by John Wiley & Sons, Ltd.

Regurgitant fraction (RF) in valvular insufficiency

	Total SV	Systemic flow volume
MR	Measure at MV	Measure at AoV
AR	Measure at AoV	Measure at PV
TR	Measure at TV	Measure at PV or AoV
PR	Measure at PV	Measure at AoV or MV

$$RF\,(\%) = 100\% \times (\text{Total } SV - \text{Systemic flow volume})/\text{Total SV}$$
$$RV\,(ml) = \text{Total SV} - \text{Systemic flow volume}$$

Mitral regurgitation

- MVP has posterior motion in mid systole on M-mode; breaks the plane of the bases by ≥ 3 mm in parasternal LAX; check for thickening, redundancy (cannot Dx in apical views).
- Coanda Effect–regurg jet hugs cardiac border, appears less severe than it really is.

Severe MR suggested
- Closure drift of the AV at the end systole in the presence of normal LVEF.
- ↑ LA/LV diameter; Flailed MV leaflet; papillary muscle rupture.
- CW: ↑↑ signal intensity/density and presence of "v" wave cut off sign.
- MV VTI/LVOT VTI ≥ 1.3.
- MR Color flow area averaged/LA Area averaged in 3 planes (mild <20%, moderate 20–40%, severe >40% mosaic part of a jet only).
- Color eccentric MR jet reaching posterior wall of LA and entering into RUPV and LUPV.
- Increased E velocity (≥ 1.4 m/sec native, >2.0 m/sec prosthetic) without increase of DT (deceleration time).

Severe MR most likely ruled out
- Presence of significant spontaneous contrast in LA.
- A > E in mitral inflow pattern.

Severe MR
- Mitral regurg volume ≥ 60 ml (mild <30 ml; moderate ≤ 59 ml).
- Regurg fraction $\geq 50\%$ (mild <30%; moderate $\leq 49\%$).
- Systolic flow reversal in at least two opposite pulmonary veins.
- MR jet reaching posterior wall of LA (mosaic part of a jet only).
- PISA radius ≥ 1 cm (aliasing velocity at 40 cm/s).

  Regurg Flow $= 2\pi r^2 V_n$ (in cm³/s).
  ERO = Regurg Flow/V_{max} (in cm²).
  Regurg Vol = ERO × VTI (in cm³);
     r = radius of PISA;
     V_n = Nyquist velocity on color;
     V_{max} = max velocity of MR on CW;
     VTI = MR envelop on CW.

- ERO ≥ 0.40 cm² (moderate 0.2–0.39 cm², mild < 0.2 cm²).
  Vena Contracta:

≥ 0.7 cm	severe MR;
0.31–0.69 cm	moderate MR;
≤ 0.3 cm	mild MR.

Pocket Guide to Echocardiography, First Edition. Andro G. Kacharava, Alexander T. Gedevanishvili, Guram G. Imnadze, Dimitri M. Tserava and Craig M. Brodsky.
© 2012 John Wiley & Sons, Ltd. Published 2012 by John Wiley & Sons, Ltd.

Following parameters suggest ↑ mean LAP in patients with ≥ moderate MR

1 Ar – A (≥ 30 ms);

2 IVRT (< 60 ms has high specificity);

3 IVRT/TE-E′ (< 3.0) may be applied for the prediction of LV filling pressures in patients with MR and normal EFs, whereas average E/E′ > 15 is applicable only in the presence of a depressed LVEF.

Aortic regurgitation

Severe AR suggested
1 Diastolic MR.
2 PISA radius > 0.7 cm with aliasing velocity at 35 cm/sec → severe AR.

	Mild	Moderate	Severe
Width jet/LVOT	<25%	25–64%	≥65%
Area jet/LVOT	<30%	30–59%	≥60%
Regurg fraction	<30%	30–49%	≥50%
Regurg volume	<30 ml	30–59 ml	≥60 mL
EROArea AI Jet	<0.1 cm²	0.1–0.29 cm²	≥0.3 cm²
Vena contracta	<0.3 cm	0.3–0.6 cm	>0.6 cm
PHT	>400 msec	200–400 msec	<200 msec
Desc aorta flow reversal	Early diastole	–	Holodiastole
CW Doppler wave signal	Faint	–	Dense

PISA method
Regurg flow $= 2\pi r^2 V_n$ (in cm³/sec).
ERO $=$ Regurg flow/V_{max} (in cm²).
Regurg vol $=$ ERO $\times$ VTI (in cm³).
  r $=$ radius of PISA;
  $V_n =$ Nyquist velocity on color;
  $V_{max} =$ max velocity of AR on CW;
  VTI $=$ AR envelop on CW.

Pocket Guide to Echocardiography, First Edition. Andro G. Kacharava, Alexander T. Gedevanishvili, Guram G. Imnadze, Dimitri M. Tsverava and Craig M. Brodsky.
© 2012 John Wiley & Sons, Ltd. Published 2012 by John Wiley & Sons, Ltd.

CHAPTER 17
Aortic stenosis

Check for:
- Valve morphology, calcification, mobility and hemodynamic severity.
- LV hypertrophy, systolic and diastolic function.
- $AVA = 0.785 \, (D_{LVOT})^2 \, (VTI_{LVOT})/(VTI_{AV})$.
- LVOT diameter in parasternal LAX, at a base of AV leaflets, during midsystole (biggest).
- VTI_{LVOT} = outflow tract (A5Ch, 1.0–1.5 cm prox to valve, with PW; avoid area of pre-stenosis flow acceleration).
- VTI_{AV} = aortic flow (A3Ch or A5Ch, at AV; use CW).
- [May use peak velocity, but VTI is preferred.].
- Gradient: peak gradient = $4v^2$ (use CW); mean gradient ≈ 2/3 peak (trace AoV VTI).
- Dimensionless index: V1/V2 < 0.25 AS is severe.
- Energy loss index (ELI) = EOA × AA/(AA–EOA) × BSA; if ≤ 0.52 cm^2/m^2 suspect severe AS.
- AoV cusp separation in M-mode: < 1.3 cm is abnormal; < 0.8 cm → suspect severe AS.

	Mean gradient	Valve area	AVA/BSA
Mild AS	<25 mmHg	>1.5 cm^2	>0.9 cm^2/m^2
Moderate AS	25–39 mmHg	1.0–1.5 cm^2	0.6–0.9 cm^2/m^2
Severe AS	≥40 mmHg	<1.0 cm^2	<0.6 cm^2/m^2

Pocket Guide to Echocardiography, First Edition. Andro G. Kacharava, Alexander T. Gedevanishvili, Guram G. Imnadze, Dimitri M. Tsverava and Craig M. Brodsky.
© 2012 John Wiley & Sons, Ltd. Published 2012 by John Wiley & Sons, Ltd.

CHAPTER 18

Recommendations for data recording and measurement for aortic stenosis

Data element	Recording	Measurement
LVOT diameter	• 2D parasternal long-axis view	• Inner edge to inner edge
	• Zoom mode	• Mid-systole
	• Adjust gain to optimize the blood tissue interface	• Parallel and adjacent to the aortic valve or at the site of velocity measurement (see text)
		• Diameter is used to calculate a circular CSA
LVOT velocity	• Pulsed-wave Doppler	• Maximum velocity from peak of dense velocity curve
	• Apical long axis or five-chamber view	• VTI traced from modal velocity
	• Sample volume positioned just on LV side of valve and moved carefuLLy into the LVOT if required to obtain laminar flow curve	
	• Velocity baseline and scale adjusted to maximize size of velocity curve	
	• Time axis (sweep speed) 100 mm/s	
	• Low wall filter setting	
	• Smooth velocity curve with a well-defined peak and a narrow velocity range at peak velocity	
AS jet velocity	• CW Doppler (dedicated transducer)	• Maximum velocity at peak of dense velocity curve
	• MuLtiple acoustic windows {e.g. apical, suprasternal, right parasternal, etc)	• Avoid noise and fine linear signals
	• Decrease gains, increase wall filter, adjust baseline, and scale to optimize signal	• VTI traced from outer edge of dense signal curve
	• Gray scaLe spectral display with expanded time scale	• Mean gradient calculated from traced velocity curve

Pocket Guide to Echocardiography, First Edition. Andro G. Kacharava, Alexander T. Gedevanishvili, Guram G. Imnadze, Dimitri M. Tsverava and Craig M. Brodsky.
© 2012 John Wiley & Sons, Ltd. Published 2012 by John Wiley & Sons, Ltd.

	• Velocity range and baseline adjusted so veLocity signal fits but fills the vertical scale	• Report window where maximum velocity obtained
Valve anatomy	• Parasternal long- and short-axis views	• Identify number of cusps in systole, raphe if present
	• Zoom mode	• Assess cusp mobility and commisural fusion
		• Assess valve calcification

CHAPTER 19

Resolution of apparent discrepancies in measures of aortic stenois severity

AS velocity >4 m/s and AVA > 1.0 cm^2

1 Check LVOT diameter measurement and compare with previous studies[a]

2 Check LVOT velocity signal for flow acceleration

3 Calculate indexed AVA when

   a Height is < 165 cm (5'5")

   b BSA < 1.5 m^2

   c BMI <22 (equivalent to 55 kg or 120 lb at this height).

4 Evaluate AR seventy

5 Evaluate for high cardiac output

   a LVOT stroke volume

   b 2D LV EF and stroke volume

Likely causes: biqh output state, moderate-severe AR, large body size

AS velocity <4 m/s and AVA < 1.0 cm^2

1 Check LVOT diameter measurement and compare with previous studies[a]

2 Check LVOT velocity signal for distance from valve

3 Calculate indexed AVA when

   a Height is < 165 cm (5'5")

   b BSA < 1.5 m^2

   c BMI <22 (equivalent to 55 kg or 120 lb at this height)

4 Evaluate for low transaortic flow volume

   a LVOT stroke volume

   b 2D LV EF and stroke volume

   c MR severity

   d Mitral stenosis

5 WhenEF < 55%

   a Assess degree of valve calcification

   b Consider dobutamine stress echocardiography

Likely causes: low cardiac output, small body size, severe MR

Pocket Guide to Echocardiography, First Edition. Andro G. Kacharava, Alexander T. Gedevanishvili, Guram G. Imnadze, Dimitri M. Tsverava and Craig M. Brodsky.
© 2012 John Wiley & Sons, Ltd. Published 2012 by John Wiley & Sons, Ltd.

CHAPTER 20

Pulmonic stenosis, pulmonic regurgitation, pulmonary hypertension

Pulmonic stenosis

	Peak PV gradient
Mild	5–35 mmHg
Moderate	36–64 mmHg or peak aortic flow velocity $\geq$ 3.0 m/s
Severe	>64 mmHg or peak aortic flow velocity > 4.0 m/s

Pulmonic Regurgitation

Severe

1 Vena contracta $\geq$75% of the RVOT;
2 PHT < 200 ms;
3 PR jet density/RVOT Systolic Jet density $\geq$ 1;
4 Holodiastolic flow reversal in MPA;
5 Mosaic part of the jet extends > 4cm from the PV to within 1 cm of TV.

Pulmonary Hypertension

- Absence of the late diastolic dip on CW Doppler of the PI jet.
- TR time $\gg$ RVOT ejection time suspect PHTN.
- RV/RA enlargement and RV hypertrophy.
- D-shaped LV (flattened septum in systole and diastole– pressure or pressure and volume overload); (flattened septum in diastole– volume overload).
- Check mitral inflow, if less than pseudonormal and no MS present, then pulm HTN is most likely not secondary to left heart problems
  RV_s pressure = TR jet maximal velocity => $(4V^2 + RA)$.
  PA_d pressure = PR jet max velocity at the end of diastole => $(4V^2 + RA)$.
- Pulmonary acceleration time (PAT) (Mahan's equation):
  $PAP_{mean} = [79 - (0.45 \times PAT)]$ (use only if HR 60–90 bpm).

	Normal	Mild	Moderate	Severe
PAT (ms)	>120	101–120	71–100	$\leq$70
PASP (mmHg)	<40	<50	<70	$\geq$70
Mean PAP (mmHg)	<25	25–34	35–44	$\geq$45

Pocket Guide to Echocardiography, First Edition. Andro G. Kacharava, Alexander T. Gedevanishvili, Guram G. Imnadze, Dimitri M. Tsverava and Craig M. Brodsky.
© 2012 John Wiley & Sons, Ltd. Published 2012 by John Wiley & Sons, Ltd.

$PAP_{mean} = 0.65 \times PASP + 0.55$ (Syyed's equation)

$PVR = TRV(m/sec)/10 \times VTI$ of $RVOT(cm) + 0.16$ (Woods Units) (Abbas's equation)

Estimation of RA pressure

RA pressure (mmHg)	IVC (cm)	IVC change c respiration
0–5	<1.7	Collapse
6–10	1.7–2.5	Decrease >50%
11–15	1.7–2.5	Decrease <50%
16–20	>2.5	Decrease <50%
>20	> 2.5	No change

CHAPTER 21

Tricuspid regurgitation and tricuspid stenosis

Tricuspid regurgitation

Leaflets visualized:
RA/RV view: Anterior, Posterior.
Apical 4-Chambers view: Anterior, Septal.

Severe TR

- RV, RA and IVC dilation.
- Visible expansion of the IVC with each systole and holosystolic reversal flow.
- Noncoaptation of TV leaflets:
  - color flow area (mosaic part of the jet) > 30% RA size and or > 10 cm^2;
  - dense CW signal with early peaking;
  - tricuspid inflow velocity > 1.0 m/s.
- Vena contracta ≥ 0.7 cm.
- PISA radius > 0.9 cm at Nyquist velocity of 50–60 cm/s.

PISA method

Regurg Flow = $2\pi r^2 V_n$ (in cm^3/s).
ERO = Regurg Flow/V_{max} (in cm^2).
Regurg Vol = ERO × VTI (in cm^3).
   r = radius of PISA;
   V_n = Nyquist velocity on color;
   V_{max} = max velocity of TR on CW;
   VTI = TR envelop on CW.

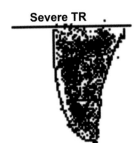
Severe TR

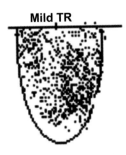
Mild TR

Figure 25 Early peaking triangular shape, late systolic concave configuration of CW signal.

Pocket Guide to Echocardiography, First Edition. Andro G. Kacharava, Alexander T. Gedevanishvili, Guram G. Imnadze, Dimitri M. Tsverava and Craig M. Brodsky.

Tricuspid stenosis

	Mean TV gradient	TVA	VTI
Mild	<2 mmHg	–	–
Moderate	2–5 mmHg	–	–
Severe	≥5 mmHg	<1 cm²	>60
Pressure half time	(**TVA = 190/PHT**)		

CHAPTER 22
Infective endocarditis

Duke Criteria
- Definite: 2 major, 1 major and 3 minor, or 5 minor.
- Possible: Fall short of above.
- Rejected: Firm alternative diagnosis.

Major
- Positive B/C (sustained bacteremia or typical organisms).
- Endocardial involvement (echo or new murmur).

Minor
- Predisposition (IVDA or structural heart dz).
- Fever > 38°C.
- Vascular phenomenon.
- Micro evidence (Cultures not meeting major criterion).
- Echo (not meeting major criterion).

Vegetation characteristics
- Echogenicity of myocardium (not calcified).
- Independent motion.
- Atrial side of MV, TV; Ventricular side of AV, PV.

When to perform TEE in patients suspected of infective endocarditis
In the following groups of patients perform **TEE**:
1 High clinical suspicion;
2 Suboptimal TTE images;
3 High risk patients: prosthetic heart valves, complex congenital heart disease, previous endocarditis, *S.aureus bacteremia*, new murmur, persistent bacteremia, evidence of embolism, new congestive heart failure;
4 High risk TTE features: large or mobile vegetations, moderate or severe valvular insufficiency, new ventricular dysfunction, suggestion of perivalvular extension;
5 Treatment failure.
  If positive treat accordingly (medical/surgical), if negative but high clinical suspicion persists, repeat TEE in 7 days, and if still negative, observe and look for other diagnosis. All other patients proceed with initial TTE, if positive treat accordingly (medical/surgical), if negative observe and look for other diagnosis.

Pocket Guide to Echocardiography, First Edition. Andro G. Kacharava, Alexander T. Gedevanishvili, Guram G. Imnadze, Dimitri M. Tserava and Craig M. Brodsky.
© 2012 John Wiley & Sons, Ltd. Published 2012 by John Wiley & Sons, Ltd.

CHAPTER 23

ACC/ASE recommendations for echocardiography in ineffective endocarditis

ACC/AHA guideline summary: Echocardiography (transthoracic [TTE] and transesophageal [TEE]) in native or prosthetic valve endocarditis (IE)

Class I – There is evidence and/or general agreement that TTE or TEE should be performed in patients with native or prosthetic valve IE in the following settings:

- TTE to detect valvular vegetations with or without positive blood cultures for the diagnosis of IE. Among patients with positive blood cultures, TEE is recommended if TTE is nondiagnostic.

- TTE to characterize the hemodynamic severity of the valve lesions in known IE. Among symptomatic patients, TEE is recommended if TTE is nondiagnostic.

- TEE as a first-line diagnostic test for prosthetic valve IE and to detect complications.

- TTE or TEE to assess complications of IE (such as abscesses, perforations, and shunts). TEE is recommended for preoperative evaluation of patients going to surgery unless the indication for surgery is apparent on TTE or imaging will delay urgent surgery.

- TTE for reassessment of high-risk patients, as defined by virulent organism, clinical deterioration, persistent or recurrent fever, a new murmur, or persistent bacteremia.

- Intraoperative TEE for patients undergoing valve surgery for IE.

Class IIa – The weight of evidence or opinion is in favor of the usefulness of TTE or TEE in patients with native or prosthetic valve IE in the following setting:

- TEE to diagnose possible IE in patients with persistent staphylococcal bacteremia who do not have a known source.

- Among patients with a prosthetic valve, TTE to diagnose IE in patients with persistent fever without bacteremia or a new murmur.

Class IIb – The weight of evidence or opinion is less well established for the usefulness of TTE or TEE in patients with native or prosthetic valve IE in the following settings:

- TEE to diagnose possible IE in patients with nosocomial staphylococcal bacteremia.

- Among patients with prosthetic valve IE, TTE for reevaluation during antibiotic therapy in the absence of signs of clinical deterioration.

Class III – There is evidence and/or general agreement that TTE is not useful in patients with native or prosthetic valve IE in the following setting:

- TTE is not indicated to reevaluate uncomplicated IE (including no valve regurgitation at baseline) during antibiotic therapy in the absence of clinical deterioration, including new physical findings, or persistent fever.

Pocket Guide to Echocardiography, First Edition. Andro G. Kacharava, Alexander T. Gedevanishvili, Guram G. Imnadze, Dimitri M. Tserava and Craig M. Brodsky.
© 2012 John Wiley & Sons, Ltd. Published 2012 by John Wiley & Sons, Ltd.

CHAPTER 24
Prosthetic valves

Bioprosthetic
Porcine (Carpentier Edwards/Hancock): have 3 struts.
Bovine pericardial.

Mechanical
Medtronic Hall/Bjork Shiley: single disc–normal to have large central jet of MR.
St. Jude: bileaflet–normal to have 3 small jets of MR.
For Prosthetic LVOT VTI/MR VTI > 0.4 excludes severe MR.
Normal prosthetic valves have small amount of regurgitation.
↑ Risk of Prosthesis-patient mismatch in AoV position when Indexed EOA = EOA prosthesis/ BSA is ≤ 0.85 cm^2/m^2; if < 0.65 cm^2/m^2 severe mismatch is likely present; ↑ Risk of Prosthesis-patient mismatch in MV position when Indexed EOA = EOA prosthesis/BSA is <1.2–1.3 cm^2/m^2.

Suspect Ao prosthesis stenosis if:
AT > 100 msec, and or AT/ET > 0.4;
MV VTI/LVOT VTI > 2.2 suspect MV prosthesis malfunction;
Increases of prosthetic MV mean TVG > 12 mmHg during Exercise SE suggests valve dysfunction or mismatch;
Increases of prosthetic AoV mean TVG > 20 mmHg during Exercise SE suggests valve dysfunction or mismatch.

Severe prosthetic AoV stenosis	Severe prosthetic MV stenosis
Mean gradient > 35 mmHg	Peak velocity ≥ 2.5 m/s
Peak velocity > 4 m/s	Mean gradient > 10 mmHg
Dimensionless index (V_1/V_2) < 0.25	MV VTI/LVOT VTI > 2.5
Acceleration time > 100 ms	EOA < 1.0 cm^2
AVA < 0.8 cm^2	PHT > 200 ms

Pocket Guide to Echocardiography, First Edition. Andro G. Kacharava, Alexander T. Gedevanishvili, Guram G. Imnadze, Dimitri M. Tsverava and Craig M. Brodsky.
© 2012 John Wiley & Sons, Ltd. Published 2012 by John Wiley & Sons, Ltd.

Severe prosthetic AoV regurgitation	Severe prosthetic MV regurgitation
Width AR jet/LVOT $\geq$65%	Vena Contracta $\geq$ 0.6 cm
Regurg Fraction >50%	Regurg Fraction > 50%
Regurg Volume >60 mL	Regurg Volume $\geq$ 60 ml
EROA AR Jet $\geq$0.3 cm^2	Jet area > 8 cm^2
Vena Contracta >0.6 cm	EROA MR Jet $\geq$ 0.5 cm^2
PHT <200 ms	CW Doppler wave signal Dense
Desc aorta flow reversal Holodiastole	
CW Doppler wave signal Dense	

CHAPTER 25

Normal echocardiographic values for prosthetic valves

Prosthetic valves in the aortic position
Normal mean gradient and area range

1. Carpentier–Edwards	14 ± 6 mmHg	1.2–3.1 cm^2
2. Hancock (stented)	11 ± 2 mmHg	1.4–2.3 cm^2;
3. Bjork –Shiley (19 mm–29 mm)	$14 \pm 3 - 31 \pm 2$ mmHg	–
4. Medtronic –Hall	12 ± 3 mmHg	–
5. Starr –Edwards	24 ± 4 mmHg	–
6. St.Jude (19 mm–31 mm)	$11 \pm 6 - 22 \pm 11$ mmHg	1.0–3.1 cm^2
7. Omniscience	14 ± 3 mmHg	–
8. Homograft	7.1 ± 3 mmHg	1.7–3.1 cm^2
9. Unstented bioprosthesis (SPV-Toronto)	4 ± 3 mmHg	1.9–2.5 cm^2
10. Mosaic 23 mm	12 ± 3 mmHg	–

Prosthetic valves in the mitral position
Normal mean gradient and area range

1. Carpentier–Edwards	6.5 ± 2.1 mmHg;	1.3–2.7 cm^2
2. Hancock (stented)	4.3 ± 2.11 mmHg;	1.6–3.5 cm^2
3. Bjork-Shiley	4.5 ± 2.0 mmHg;	1.6–3.7 cm^2
4. Medtronic–Hall	3.1 ± 0.9 mmHg;	1.5–3.9 cm^2
5. Starr–Edwards	4.6 ± 2.4 mmHg;	1.2–2.5 cm^2
6. St.Jude	4.5 ± 2.0 mmHg;	1.8–4.4 cm^2
7. OmniScience	3.3 ± 0.9 mmHg;	1.6–3.1 cm^2

Annular rings in the mitral position
Normal mean gradient and area range

1. Carpentier–Edwards	3.8 ± 0.4	1.8–3.8 cm^2
2. Duran	3.8 ± 1.1	1.9–3.9 cm^2

Pocket Guide to Echocardiography, First Edition. Andro G. Kacharava, Alexander T. Gedevanishvili, Guram G. Imnadze, Dimitri M. Tserava and Craig M. Brodsky.
© 2012 John Wiley & Sons, Ltd. Published 2012 by John Wiley & Sons, Ltd.

Important info when evaluating pt with prosthetic valve include:
1 Reason;
2 Type and size;
3 Date of surgery;
4 Blood pressure and heart rate at the time of exam;
5 Height, weight and BSA of the patient.

CHAPTER 26
Congenital heart disease

VSD
Muscular
Central Inlet VSD seen in 4-chambers view (upper 1/3 VS) and in subcostal 4-chambers view (upper 1/3 VS).
Infracristal Inlet VSD seen in (lower 2/3 VS) in apical 4-chambers also in 3-chambers and 5-chambers views; also seen in subcostal 4-chamber (lower 2/3 VS).
Supracristal Outlet VSD seen in SAX AoV view jet directed toward the RVOT and PV.

Membranous
Perimembranous inlet VSD (SAX AoV jet is seen under the TV) and perimembranous outlet subaortic VSD (5-chambers apical or subcostal views jet is seen under under the AoV).

ASD
Ostium secundum: most common.
Ostium primum: associated with membran. VSD, AV canal defect, cleft MV.
Sinus venosus: associated with anomalous PV drainage (RUPV in 80–90%).
Roofless coronary sinus: associated with anomalous L SVC.

Tetralogy of Fallot: RVH, PS, VSD, overriding aorta.
PDA: desc aorta → main PA (near left PA).
Aortic Coarctation: assoc c bicuspid AV.
l-TGA: congenitally corrected (PV → RV → Ao; VC's → LV → PA).
d-TGA: not corrected (PV → LV → PA; VC's → RV → Ao).
Ebstein's: apical displacement of TV; assoc c ASD or PFO, WPW.

Shunt ratios (Qp/Qs)
ASD – measure Qp at PV or TV, and Qs at AV or MV.
VSD – measure Qp at PV or MV, and Qs at AV or TV.
PDA – measure Qp at AV or MV, and Qs at PV or TV.

Pocket Guide to Echocardiography, First Edition. Andro G. Kacharava, Alexander T. Gedevanishvili, Guram G. Imnadze, Dimitri M. Tsverava and Craig M. Brodsky.
© 2012 John Wiley & Sons, Ltd. Published 2012 by John Wiley & Sons, Ltd.

CHAPTER 27
Miscellaneous

- Eustachian valve: redundant endocardial ridge in RA by IVC.
- Chiari network: remnant of the sinus venosus, present in 2–3% of normal adults; thin, weblike membrane c̄ multiple fenestrations, from IVC to septum, mobile.
- Atrial septal aneurysm: Excursion ≥ 15 mm.
- Lipomatous hypertrophy: bilobed appearance, > 15 mm thick.
- Coronary sinus: parasternal long is best view; posterior and superior to MV; dilated with increased RA pressure, persistant L-SVC, unroofed coronary sinus.

Pocket Guide to Echocardiography, First Edition. Andro G. Kacharava, Alexander T. Gedevanishvili, Guram G. Imnadze, Dimitri M. Tsverava and Craig M. Brodsky.
© 2012 John Wiley & Sons, Ltd. Published 2012 by John Wiley & Sons, Ltd.

CHAPTER 28
Aortic diseases

Aortic atherosclerosis (Katz's classification)

Grade I   Normal.
Grade II   Atherosclerosis: intimal thickening $\geq$ 3 mm.
Grade III   Atherosclerosis: prothruding plaque < 4 mm.
Grade IV*   Atherosclerosis: protruding plaque $\geq$ 4 mm.
Grade V*   Atherosclerosis: mobile, ulcerated plaque $\geq$ 4 mm.

*Grades IV, V associated with increased embolic risk.

Aortic Dissection: tear in intima and media extending down the aorta +/− branch vessels. The intimal flap separates the false lumen from the true lumen of the aorta.
- True lumen–may be smaller, but exhibits systolic expansion.
- False lumen–may have thrombus or swirling flow.

Intramural hematoma: dissection w/o intimal tear; no communication between true and false lumens. Intimal surface is smooth; hematoma is > 7 mm thick. Note increased aortic wall thickness with pockets of lucency.

Penetrating aortic ulcer: bleeding into an atherosclerotic plaque through the aortic intima.

Traumatic aortic injury: 2° to blunt trauma; often caused by a deceleration injury. The majority of tears are located at the isthmus of the descending aorta, at the location of the ligamentum arteriosum (aortic transection).

Pocket Guide to Echocardiography, First Edition. Andro G. Kacharava, Alexander T. Gedevanishvili, Guram G. Imnadze, Dimitri M. Tsverava and Craig M. Brodsky.
© 2012 John Wiley & Sons, Ltd. Published 2012 by John Wiley & Sons, Ltd.

CHAPTER 29

Indication for surgery in aortic diseases

The indications for surgery for thoracic aneurysm include:
- The presence of symptoms.
- A diameter of 50 to 60 mm for an ascending aortic aneurysm and 60 to 70 mm for a descending aortic aneurysm; often ≥70 mm in high risk patients.
- Accelerated growth rate (≥5 mm per year) in aneurysms.
- Evidence of TypeA dissection.

The indications for surgery for abdominal aneurysm include:

In a consensus statement of the Society for Vascular Surgery, the American Association of Vascular Surgery, and the Society for Vascular Medicine and Biology, the following schedule was recommended for abdominal aneurysm:
- The presence of symptoms— referral to a vascular specialist;
- Aortic diameter <3 cm — no further testing;
- Aneurysm 3 to 4 cm — annual ultrasound;
- Aneurysm 4 to 4.5 cm — ultrasound every six months;
- Aneurysm > 4.5 cm — referral to a vascular specialist.

Carefully selected patients may benefit from early surgery at an aneurysm diameter of 4.5 to 5.0 cm. This is most applicable to women who have a four-fold higher rate of rupture than men and are at risk for rupture at smaller aneurysm diameters. Patients with an aneurysm that expands more than 0.5 cm within a six month interval, grows to ≥ 5.5 cm, or becomes symptomatic should undergo elective repair.

Pocket Guide to Echocardiography, First Edition. Andro G. Kacharava, Alexander T. Gedevanishvili, Guram G. Imnadze, Dimitri M. Tsverava and Craig M. Brodsky.

CHAPTER 30

Transthoracic echocardiographic and Doppler protocols for assessment of ventricular dyssynchrony

Two methods of diagnosing cardiac intraventricular dyssynchrony with tissue Doppler imaging

1 The asynchrony index

  A Measure of the standard deviation of time to peak systolic velocity of 12 LV segments (6 basal and 6 middle) in the 3 standard apical views (2-, 3-, 4-chambers views). Time to peak systolic velocity is measured from the beginning of "q" wave of the QRS complex on the ECG. Ts-SD of ≥ 31.4 msec had a sensitivity of 87% and specificity 81% for intraventricular dyssynchrony.

  B Simplified method to measure asynchrony: Measure maximal difference between peak systolic velocities of any 2 of the 12 above mentioned segments. A value > 100 msec indicates dyssynchrony.

2 Septal to lateral wall delay

  Measure difference of time to peak systolic velocity between basal septal and lateral walls. A value > 65 msec indicates dyssynchrony and has a sensitivity and specificity of 80% to predict response to CRT.

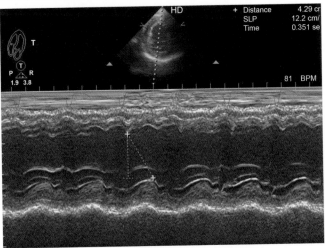

Figure 26 Diagnosing cardiac intraventricular dyssynchrony.

Pocket Guide to Echocardiography, First Edition. Andro G. Kacharava, Alexander T. Gedevanishvili, Guram G. Imnadze, Dimitri M. Tsverava and Craig M. Brodsky.

Antero-septal wall to Infero-lateral wall systolic time delay ≥ 130 msec indicates of intraventricular dyssynchrony (SAX view).

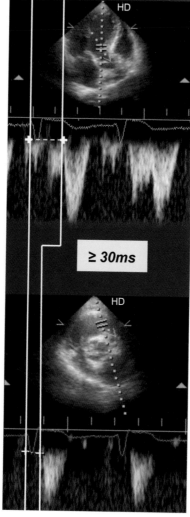

Figure 27 Diagnosing cardiac interventricular dyssynchrony.

Delay of ≥ 30 msec in Aortic systolic flow onset, compared to pulmonic systolic flow onset indicates interventricular dyssynchrony.

CHAPTER 31

Indications, contraindications and complications of transesophageal echocardiographic examination

Indications for TEE

1 Cardiac or aortic source of emboli.
2 Congenital heart disease/intracardiac shunts.
3 Endocarditis (moderate/high clinical suspicion or initial risk).
4 Cardiac tumors/masses.
5 Aortic diseases (dissection, aneurysm/transsection/ulcer/hematoma).
6 Valvular prosthesis malfunction.
7 Pre a.fib/flutter cardioversion/ablation.
8 Mechanism of regurgitation in native valves.
9 Inadequate TTE images.
10 Correct position of IABP.
11 Mitral valve examination pre and post repair.
12 Pre and post- mitral valve valvuloplasty.
13 Intraop evaluation.

Contraindication
Absolute
1 Uncooperative or unwilling patient.
2 Esophageal obstruction/stricture/tumor.
3 Esophageal diverticulum.
4 Perforated viscus.
5 Recent Esophageal or gastric surgery.
6 Instability of the cervical spine.
7 Active upper GI bleeding.

Relative
1 Nonbleeding esophageal varices.
2 Severe cervical arthritis.
3 Significant oropharyngeal distortion.
4 Severe cardiopulmonary distress.
5 Extreme oropharyngeal muscle weakness.
6 Severe coagulopathy (INR > 5.0; PTT > 100 sec, Platelets < 25000).

Pocket Guide to Echocardiography, First Edition. Andro G. Kacharava, Alexander T. Gedevanishvili, Guram G. Imnadze, Dimitri M. Tsverava and Craig M. Brodsky
© 2012 John Wiley & Sons, Ltd. Published 2012 by John Wiley & Sons, Ltd.

Complications

1 Pharyngeal, esophageal, gastric laceration/perforation.
2 Lip or dental injury, parotid gland swelling.
3 Upper GI bleeding/Hematemesis.
4 Thermal, electrical, or chemical burn.
5 Dysphagia or odynophagia.
6 Vocal cord injury/paralysis.
7 Hypertension/hypotension.
8 Arrhythmias/MI/Death.
9 Vomiting/aspiration/Bronchospasm/laryngospasm.
10 Hypoxemia/upper airway obstruction/respiratory arrest.
11 Ruptured aortic aneurysm/dissection.
12 Methemglobinemia.

Important points

1 To reverse Benzo use flumazenil 0.2 mg i.v. max total dose 1.0 mg.
2 To reverse narcotic analgesic effect use naloxone 0.4 mg i.v. every 2 min up to max total dose 10 mg.
3 To treat methemglobinemia give methylene blue 1 mg/kg 1% solution i.v. over 5 min, up to total maximal dose 7 mg/kg.

CHAPTER 32

Routine approach to any transesophageal echocardiographic and recommended views for evaluation of aorta

Routine approach to any TEE view

1 Obtain gross view without color, Doppler or Magnification.
2 Place color Doppler over the individual structure.
3 Doppler the available jets if feasible.
4 Magnify the view to better review the suspected pathology.
5 Move to another view.

Recommended tomographic views in TEE evaluation of the aorta

1 The midesophageal AoV short axis view.
2 The midesophageal AoV long axis view.
3 The upper esophageal ascendic aortic short axis view.
4 The upper esophageal ascendic aortic long axis view.
5 The upper esophageal aortic arch short axis view.
6 The upper esophageal aortic arch long axis view.
7 The descending aortic short axis view at the level of isthmus.
8 The descending aortic long axis view at the level of isthmus.
9 The descending aortic short axis view.
10 The descending aortic long axis view.

Pocket Guide to Echocardiography, First Edition. Andro G. Kacharava, Alexander T. Gedevanishvili, Guram G. Imnadze, Dimitri M. Tsverava and Craig M. Brodsky.
© 2012 John Wiley & Sons, Ltd. Published 2012 by John Wiley & Sons, Ltd.

Terminology used to describe manipulation of the probe and transducer during image acquisition

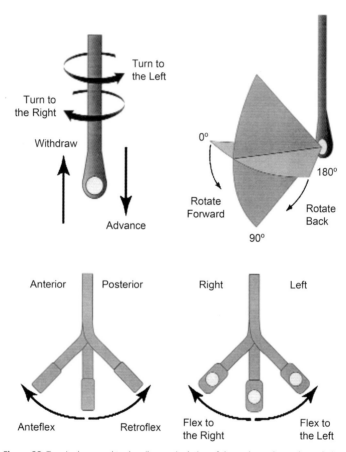

Figure 28 Terminology used to describe manipulation of the probe and transducer during image acquisition. (Reproduced, with permission, from Shanewise, et al., 1999.)

Pocket Guide to Echocardiography, First Edition. Andro G. Kacharava, Alexander T. Gedevanishvili, Guram G. Imnadze, Dimitri M. Tsverava and Craig M. Brodsky.
© 2012 John Wiley & Sons, Ltd. Published 2012 by John Wiley & Sons, Ltd.

CHAPTER 34
Diagrams of standard transesophageal echocardiographic views

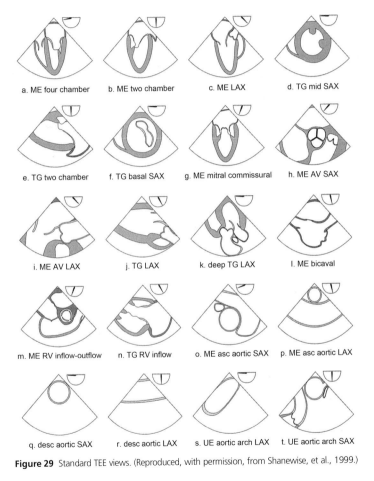

Figure 29 Standard TEE views. (Reproduced, with permission, from Shanewise, et al., 1999.)

Pocket Guide to Echocardiography, First Edition. Andro G. Kacharava, Alexander T. Gedevanishvili, Guram G. Imnadze, Dimitri M. Tsverava and Craig M. Brodsky.

Transesophageal echocardiographic measurements

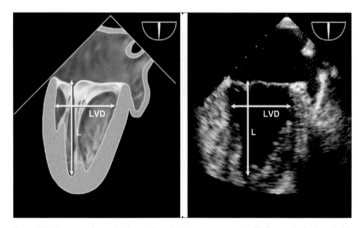

Figure 30 Transesophageal echocardiographic measurements of left ventricular length (L) and minor diameter (LVD) from midesophageal 2-chambers view, usually best imaged at multiplane angle of approximately 60 to 90 degrees. (Reproduced, with permission, from Lang et al., 2005.)

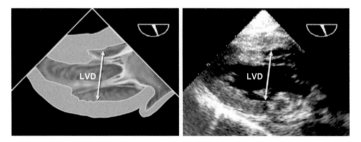

Figure 31 Transesophageal echocardiographic measurements of left ventricular (LV) minor-axis diameter (LVD) from transgastricric 2-chambers view of LV, usually best imaged at angle of approximately 90 to 110 degrees after optimizing maximum obtainable LV size by adjustment of medial-lateral rotation. (Reproduced, with permission, from Lang et al., 2005.)

Pocket Guide to Echocardiography, First Edition. Andro G. Kacharava, Alexander T. Gedevanishvili, Guram G. Imnadze, Dimitri M. Tsverava and Craig M. Brodsky.
© 2012 John Wiley & Sons, Ltd. Published 2012 by John Wiley & Sons, Ltd.

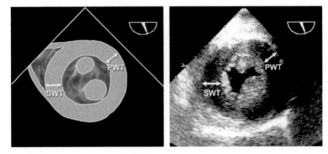

Figure 32 Transesophageal echocardiographic measurements of wall thickness of left ventricular (LV) septal wall (SWT) and posterior wall (PWT) from transgastric short axis view of LV, at papillary muscle level, usually best imaged at angle of approximately 0 to 30 degrees. (Reproduced, with permission, from Lang et al., 2005.)

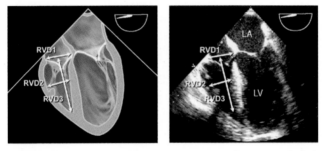

Figure 33 Transesophageal echocardiographic measurements of right ventricular (RV) diameters from midesophageal 4-chambers view, best imaged after optimizing maximum obtainable rv size by varying angles from approximately 0 to 20 degrees. (Reproduced, with permission, from Lang et al., 2005.)

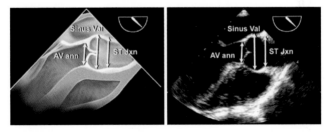

Figure 34 Measurement of aortic root diameters at aortic valve annulus (AV ann) level, sinuses of Valsalva (Sinus Val), and sinotubular junction (ST Jxn) from midesophageal long-axis view of aortic valve, usually at angle of approximately 110 to 150 degrees. Annulus is measured by convention at base of aortic leaflets. although leading edge to leading edge technique is demonstrated for the Sinus Val and ST Jxn, Some prefer inner edge to inner edge method. (Reproduced, with permission, from Lang, et al., 2005.)

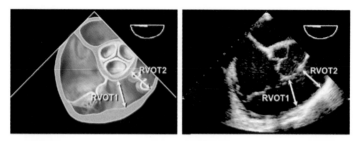

Figure 35 Measurement of right ventricular outflow tract diameter at subpulmonary region (RVOT1) and pulmonic valve annulus (RVOT2) in midesophageal aortic valve short-axis view, using multiplane angle of approximately 45 to 70 degrees. (Reproduced, with permission, from Lang, et al., 2005.)

CHAPTER 36

Transesophageal echocardiographic diagram of the regional blood supply to cardiac wall segments

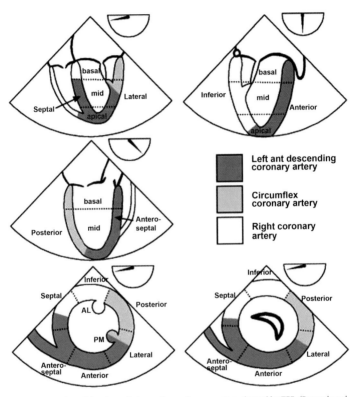

Figure 36 Regional blood supply to cardiac wall segments evaluated by TEE. (Reproduced, with permission, from Sidebotham, et al., 2003.)

Pocket Guide to Echocardiography, First Edition. Andro G. Kacharava, Alexander T. Gedevanishvili, Guram G. Imnadze, Dimitri M. Tsverava and Craig M. Brodsky.
© 2012 John Wiley & Sons, Ltd. Published 2012 by John Wiley & Sons, Ltd.

CHAPTER 37

Transesophageal echocardiographic orientation for assessment of the mitral valve

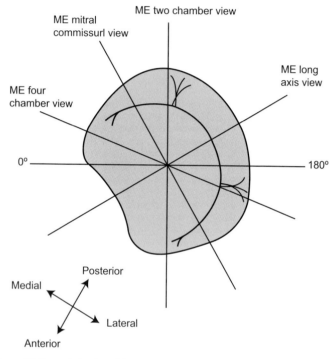

Figure 37 Short axis drawing of the mitral valve illustrating how it is transected by mid esophageal views. rotating from multiplane angle from 0 degrees to 180 degrees moves the imaging plane axially through the entire mitral valve. (Reproduced, with permission, from Shanewise, et al., 1999.)

Pocket Guide to Echocardiography, First Edition. Andro G. Kacharava, Alexander T. Gedevanishvili, Guram G. Imnadze, Dimitri M. Tsverava and Craig M. Brodsky.
© 2012 John Wiley & Sons, Ltd. Published 2012 by John Wiley & Sons, Ltd.

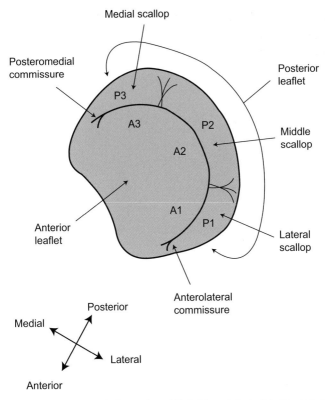

Figure 38 Anatomy of mitral valve. A1, lateral third of the anterior leaflet; A2, middle third of the anterior leaflet; A3, medial third of the anterior leaflet; P1, lateral scallop of the posterior leaflet; P2, middle scallop of the posterior leaflet; P3, medial scallop of the posterior leaflet. (Reproduced, with permission, from Shanewise, et al., 1999.)

CHAPTER 38
Diagrams of transesophageal echocardiographic views in the evaluation of the mitral valve

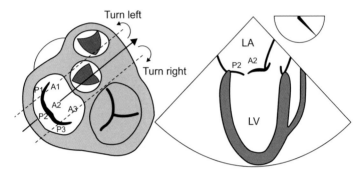

Figure 39 Midesophageal 3-chambers view for evaluation of the mitral valve. (Reproduced, with permission, from Sidebotham et al., 2003.)

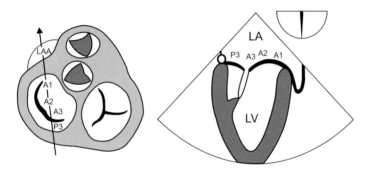

Figure 40 Midesophageal 2-chambers view for evaluation of the mitral valve. (Reproduced, with permission, from Sidebotham et al., 2003.)

Pocket Guide to Echocardiography, First Edition. Andro G. Kacharava, Alexander T. Gedevanishvili, Guram G. Imnadze, Dimitri M. Tsverava and Craig M. Brodsky.
© 2012 John Wiley & Sons, Ltd. Published 2012 by John Wiley & Sons, Ltd.

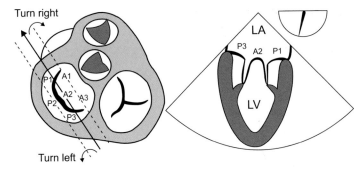

Figure 41 Midesophageal commissural view for evaluation of the mitral valve. (Reproduced, with permission, from Sidebotham et al., 2003.)

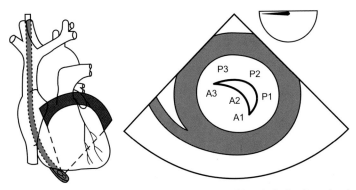

Figure 42 Transgastric basal short axis view for evaluation of the mitral valve. (Reproduced, with permission, from Sidebotham et al., 2003.)

CHAPTER 39

References and Recommended Literature

Baumgartner H, et al. Echocardiographic assessment of valve stenosis: EAE/ASE Recommendations for Clinical Practice. *J Am Soc Echocardiogr* 2009; **22**: 1–23.

Dal-Bianco JP, et al. Role of echocardiography in the diagnosis of constrictive pericarditis. *J Am Soc Echocardiogr* 2009; **22**: 24–33.

Feigenbaum H. *Echocardiography*, 6th edn. Philadelphia: Lea & Febiger, 2005.

Horton KD, et al. Assessment of the Right Ventricle by Echocardiography: A Primer for Cardiac Sonographers. *J Am Soc Echocardiogr* 2009; **22**: 776–792.

Kerut EK, McIlwain EF, Plotnick GD. *Handbook of Echo-Doppler Interpretation*, 2nd edn. Blackwell/Futura, 2002.

Lang RM, et al. Recommendations for Chamber Quantification: A Report from the American Society of Echocardiography's Guidelines and Standards Committee and the Chamber Quantification Writing Group, Developed in Conjunction with the European Association of Echocardiography, a Branch of the European Society of Cardiology. *J Am Soc Echocardiogr* 2005; **18**: 1440–1463.

Nagueh SF, et al. Recommendations for Evaluation of Left Ventricular Diastolic Function by Echocardiography. *J Am Soc Echocardiogr* 2009; **22**: 107–133.

Oh JK, Seward JB, Tajik AJ. *The Echo Manual*, 3rd edn. Philadelphia: Lippincott Williams & Wilkins, 2006.

Otto CM. *Textbook of Clinical Echocardiography*, 3rd edn. Philadelphia: Saunders, 2005.

Pellikka PA, et al. American Society of Echocardiography Recommendations for Performance, Interpretation, and Application of Stress Echocardiography. *J Am Soc Echocardiogr* 2007; **20**: 1021–1041.

Perrino AC, Reeves ST. *A Practical Approach to Transesophageal Echocardiography*. Philadelphia: Lippincott Williams & Wilkins, 2003.

Roelandt JRTC, Pandian NG. *Multiplane Transesophageal Echocardiography*. Churchill Livingstone, 1996.

Rudski LG. Guidelines for the Echocardiographic Assessment of the Right Heart in Adults: a report from the American Society of Echocardiography endorsed by the European Association of Echocardiography (a registered branch of the European Society of Cardiology and the Canadian Society of Echocardiography. *J Am Soc Echocardiogr* 2010; **23**: 685–713.

Savage RM, Aronson S, *Comprehensive Textbook of Intraoperative Transesophageal Echocardiography*. Philadelphia: Lippincott Williams & Wilkins, 2005.

Shanewise JS, et al. ASE/SCA Guidelines for Performing a Comprehensive Intraoperative Multiplane Transesophageal Echocardiography Examination: Recommendations of the American Society of Echocardiography Council for Intraoperative Echocardiography and the Society of Cardiovascular Anesthesiologists Task Force for Certification in Perioperative Transesophageal Echocardiography. *J Am Soc Echocardiogr* 1999; **12**: 884–900.

Sidebotham D, Merry A, Legget M. *Practical Perioperative Transoesophageal Echocardiography*, London, UK: Butterworth-Henemann, 2003.

Weyman AE. *Principles and Practice of Echocardiography*, 2nd edn. Philadelphia: Lea & Febiger, 1994.

Zoghbi WA, et al. Recommendations for Evaluation of Prosthetic Valves with Echocardiography and Doppler Ultrasound. A report from the American Society of Echocardiography's Guidelines and Standards Committee and the Task Force on Prosthetic Valves, developed in conjunction with the American College of Cardiology Cardiovascular Imaging Committee, the Cardiac Imaging Committee of the American Heart Association, the European Association of Echocardiography

Pocket Guide to Echocardiography, First Edition. Andro G. Kacharava, Alexander T. Gedevanishvili, Guram G. Imnadze, Dimitri M. Tserava and Craig M. Brodsky.

© 2012 John Wiley & Sons, Ltd. Published 2012 by John Wiley & Sons, Ltd.

(a registered branch of the European Society of Cardiology), the Japanese Society of Echocardiography, and the Canadian Society of Echocardiography. Endorsed by the American College of Cardiology Foundation, the American Heart Association, the European Association of Echocardiography, the Japanese Society of Echocardiography, and the Canadian Society of Echocardiography. *J Am Soc Echocardiogr* 2009; **22**: 975–1014.

Zoghbi WA, et al. Recommendations for Evaluation of the Severity of Native Valvular Regurgitation with Two-Dimensional and Doppler Echocardiography. *J Am Soc Echocardiogr* 2003; **16**: 777–802.

Supplement to

Pocket Guide of Echocardiography

Andro G. Kacharava MD, PhD

Echocardiography Laboratory
Emory University School of Medicine
Atlanta VA Medical Center
Atlanta, GA, USA

Alexander T. Gedevanishvili, MD

Echocardiography Laboratory
Southern CardioPulmonary Associates
West Georgia Health System
LaGrange, GA, USA

Guram G. Imnadze, MD, PhD

Schuechtermann Klinik,
Bad Rothenfelde, Germany

Dimitri M. Tsverava, MD

Tbilisi Medical Academy
MediClubGeorgia
Tbilisi, Georgia

Craig M. Brodsky, MD

Echocardiography Laboratory
Boca Raton Community Hospital
Boca Raton, FL, USA

Comprehensive TTE examination

1st: 2-D parasternal long-axis view

1 Zoom and measure LVOT diameter on still frame during mid to late systole.

2 Note presence of spontaneous contrast in RV, AO, LV, or LA.

3 Note presence of a mass in RV, AO, LV, or LA.

4 Characterize mass (zoom on it if needed):
1. shape; 2. mobility; 3. size; 4. attachment site.

5 Check aortic wall thickness and presence of calcification.

6 Check for a proximal aortic dissection (presence of double lumen and intimal flap), ascending aortic aneurysm, and aortic root abscess.

7 Note presence of a mass on aortic and/or mitral valves.

8 Characterize mass (zoom on it if needed):
1. shape; 2. mobility; 3. size; 4. attachment site.

9 Note size of coronary sinus (normal < 1.5 cm).

10 Characterize LV wall segments (antero-septal: basal and mid; inferolateral: basal and mid):
1. Thickness 2. Motion – normal vs:
a. hypokinesis; b. akinesis; c. dyskinesis.

11 Note presence of an aneurysm, pseudoaneurysm and intramyocardial dissecting hematoma.

12 Note decreased amplitude of systolic aortic cusp motion due to:
A. sclerosis/stenosis; B. calcification; C. decreased stroke volume. D. HOCM;
E. supra- and subvalvular stenosis

13 Note presence of doming, prolapse and flail of aortic valve cusps.

14 Note decreased amplitude of diastolic mitral valve leaflets opening due to:
A. stenosis; B. decreased stroke volume.

15 Note presence of pericardial effusion, location and qualitatively assess size:
A. anterior; B. posterior; C. circumferential.

16 Check for signs of cardiac tamponade: A. late diastolic and early systolic collapse of LA;
B. early diastolic collapse of the RV.

17 Check for presence of thickened and calcified pericardium.

18 Check for presence of intrapericardial mass. Characterize it:
1. shape; 2. mobility; 3. size; 4. attachment site.

19 Note calcification and its severity of mitral annulus:
1. mild; 2. moderate; 3. severe.

20 Check for the presence of mitral or aortic valve abscess.

21 Note mitral valve calcification, thickening, mobility, subvalvular thickening (Assign points and assess mitral valve score). "Hockey Stick" sign in mitral stenosis.

22 Note mitral valve prolapse and/or flail: anterior; posterior; both leaflets.

23 Note presence of chordal and/or posterior-medial pap muscle rupture.

24 Note presence of restricted motion of the MV leaflets.

Pocket Guide to Echocardiography, First Edition. Andro G. Kacharava, Alexander T. Gedevanishvili, Guram G. Imnadze, Dimitri M. Tsverava and Craig M. Brodsky.

© 2012 John Wiley & Sons, Ltd. Published 2012 by John Wiley & Sons, Ltd.

25 Note presence of a posterior-medial papillary muscle dysfunction.

26 Note presence of prosthetic valve in aortic position and/or in mitral position.

Characterize valve:

Type of Valve	
Bioprosthetic	**Mechanical**
Carpentier-Edwards	St. Jude
Hancock	Bjork-Shiley
Other	Starr-Edwards
	Medtronic-Hall
	Other

27 Stability of the prosthetic valve sitting and absence of rocking.

28 Note presence of a mass on aortic and/or mitral prosthetic valves.

29 Characterize mass (zoom on it if needed):

1. shape; 2. mobility; 3. size; 4. attachment site.

30 Check for presence of a MV annular abscess.

31 Note presence of annuloplasty ring.

2nd: 2-D color Doppler in parasternal long-axis view

1 Note presence of the Aortic Regurgitation (AR).

2 Characterize and assess severity of the AR jet:

  a Measure width of the AR jet and calculate jet/LVOT diameter ratio.

  b Measure width of the AR jet area and calculate jet/LVOT area ratio.

  c Measure width of the vena contracta of the AR jet.

  d Comment on eccentricity and direction of the AR jet.

  (See the AR severity assessment in this book.)

3 Note presence of the Mitral Regurgitation (MR).

4 Characterize and assess severity of the MR jet:

  a Comment on eccentricity and direction of the MR jet.

  b Comment on length (mosaic part only) of MR jet (reaching posterior wall of LA).

  c Measure width of the vena contracta of the MR jet.

  d Measure width of the MR jet area (mosaic part only) and calculate jet/LA area ratio.

  (See the MR severity assessment in this book.)

5 Check the color flow of blood in the dissecting septal or posterior wall intramyocardial hematoma if present.

6 Check the color flow of blood in the posterior wall pseudoaneurysm if present.

7 Check for aliasing (high velocity) diastolic color flow of the blood through the MV inflow (suspect MV obstruction).

8 Check for aliasing (high velocity) systolic color flow of the blood through the LV outflow tract (suspect HOCM, Subvalvular stenosis) or intracavitary obstruction.

9 Check for presence of Ventricular Septal Defect (VSD) color jet in systole from LV to RV, or from LV to RA in Gerbode defect.

10 Check for presence of color flow of the blood in proximal Aortic Dissection false lumen.

11 Check for presence of the perivalvular leak through Aoritc and Mitral valves in the presence of AV and MV prosthesis.

12 Check for presence of Aortic Root and/or MV annulus communicating abscess cavity.

13 Differentiate between LV diverticulum and aneurysm based on color flow in and out of the cavity during systole and diastole (flow into the cavity during systole in the presence of aneurysm).

14 Check for the presence of MV leaflet and or Aortic valve cusp perforation.

3rd: M-mode scan in parasternal long view

1 Measure Aortic Root size at the level of:

  a Aortic sinuses.

  b Sinotubular junction.

  c Proximal ascending aorta.

2 Measure LA diameter and define severity of LA dilation if present.

3 Note sclerosis and calcification of Aortic Walls

4 Note shape and distance of right and Noncoronary Aortic valve cusps separation.

  a Quadrangular (normal).

  b Trapezoid (low stroke volume beat).

  c Triangular (low stroke volume beat).

  d <0.7 cm (suggests presence of a significant aortic stenosis).

  e Midsystolic notching (suggests dynamic LVOT or intracavitary obstruction).

5 Note coaptation line of the right and noncoronary cusps

  a. midline (normal); b. eccentric (could be sign of the bicuspid aortic valve).

6 Note the high frequency fluttering of the aortic valve right and noncoronary cusps during systole (can be suggestive of increased flow through the valve).

  1. Note amplitude of the aortic root motion and presence of flattening of the posterior wall of the aorta (suggests low stroke volume).

7 Note presence of spontaneous contrast in aorta and LA.

8 Note presence of a mass in aortic root and/or aortic valve cusps and if present characterize it:

  1. mobility; 2. size; 3. site of attachment.

9 Note presence of a mass in LA and if present characterize it:

  1. mobility; 2. size; 3. site of attachment.

10 Note presence of a mass in RV cavity and if present characterize it:

  1. mobility, 2, size, 3. site of attachment.

11 Check for the presence of anterior and posterior pericardial effusion.

12 Check for presence of thickened and calcified pericardium (suspect constrictive pericarditis in appropriate clinical setting).

13 Check the RV size and wall motion.

14 Check for the presence of the RV early diastolic collapse (if present, suspect cardiac tamponade).

15 Note MV leaflets thickening and mobility.

16 Check for presence of LA late diastolic early systolic collapse (if present, suspect cardiac tamponade).

17 Check for the presence of systolic anterior motion (SAM) with Valsalva maneuver (if present, suspect HOCM).

18 Measure "E" to "S" separation distance (>2.5 cm suggests LVEF <25%).

19 Check for the presence of mitral valve prolapse (MVP) with Valsalva maneuver.

20 Check for the presence of anterior motion of the posterior leaflet, and flattening of the E-F slope (if present, suspect mitral stenosis).

21 Measure basal and mid antero-septal LVED wall diameter and assess mobility and its thickening during systole.

22 Measure basal and mid inferolateral LVED wall diameter and assess mobility and its thickening during systole.
23 Measure LVESD and LVEDD.
24 Measure intraventricular dyssynchrony (septal–posterior wall delay), if present.
25 Color M-mode through AV and MV to assess presence of AI and MR (this is optional).
26 Color Doppler tissue M-mode to better assess thickness and mobility of the LV walls basal and mid antero–septal and inferolateral segments.

4th: 2-D RA/RV inflow view

1 Comment on anterior and posterior leaflets of tricuspid valve:
A. mobility; B. coaptation; C. doming; D. prolapse. E. Flail; F. Thickness and Calcification.
2 Note presence of spontaneous contrast in RV, and/or RA.
3 Note presence of a mass in RV, and/or RA.
4 Characterize the mass if present:
1. shape; 2. mobility; 3. size; 4. attachment site.
5 Note presence of tricuspid annulus calcification.
6 Note presence of Eustachian valve and Chiari network.
7 Note presence of mass on tricuspid valve.
8 Characterize the mass if present on the tricuspid valve:
1. shape; 2. mobility; 3. size; 4. attachment site.
9 Check for the presence of tricuspid valve and/or annular abscess.
10 Note presence of segmental wall motion abnormalities of the RV.
11 Note presence of McConnell sign (RV apex contracts well, but the rest of the RV is dilated and poorly contracts) (if present, suspect acute pressure overload of the RV).
12 Note presence of a pericardial effusion.
13 Note early diastolic collapse of RV and late diastolic early systolic collapse of RA (if present suspect cardiac tamponade).
14 Note presence of "spontaneous contrast" in RA and/or RV.
15 Note presence of TV prosthesis.
16 Characterize TV prosthesis:
 A Type: 1. bioprosthetic; 2. mechanical.
 B Rocking motion (if present suggests dehiscence).
 C Mass: 1. shape; 2. mobility; 3. size; 4. attachment site.
 D Leaflet thickness.
17 Note presence of pacemaker/ICD/catheter in RA and RV.
18 Note presence of annuloplasty ring.
19 Note TV calcification, thickening, mobility, subvalvular thickening.
20 Note TV prolapse and/or flail: Anterior; Posterior; both leaflets.
21 Note decreased amplitude of diastolic tricuspid valve leaflets opening due to: A. stenosis; B. decreased stroke volume.

5th: 2-D RA/RV inflow view color Doppler view

1 Note presence of TR jet.
2 Characterize the TR jet if present:
A. Eccentric, B. Central.
3 Assess severity of the TR jet by measuring:
 A Vena contracta.
 B PISA method for ERO calculation.
 C Mosaic color flow area/RA area ratio.
   (See the TR severity assessment in this book).

4 Note presence of periprosthetic and intravalvular TR jets.
5 Note presence of perforated TV leaflet.

6th: 2-D RA/RV view PW and CW Doppler view

1 Measure TR max velocity using CW Doppler and calculate RV/RA gradient.
2 Assess TV inflow pattern with PW Doppler:
  A Impaired relaxation.
  B Pseudonormal.
  C Restrictive.
  (See diastolic function assessment in this book).
3 Assess respiratory variation of TV inflow velocity (if significant variation present suspect pathology).
4 Measure TV maximal inflow blood velocity with CW Doppler.
5 Measure TV mean gradient if TS suspected.
6 TR jet density and shape to be noted to assess severity of TR.
  (See the TR severity assessment in this book.)

7th: Parasternal 2-D short axis view through the aortic valve

  1 Comment on tricuspid valve leaflets:
  A. structure; B. mobility; C. thickness, D. calcification; E. coaptation; F. flail and prolapse.
  2 Note presence of the tricuspid valve annular calcification.
  3 Note presence of RV and/or RA and/or LA mass.
  4 Characterize the mass if present:
  1. shape; 2. mobility; 3. size; 4. attachment site.
  5 Note presence of Eustachian valve and Chiari network.
  6 Note presence of tricuspid valve mass and characterize it if present:
  1. shape; 2. mobility; 3. size; 4. attachment site.
  7 Check for the presence of tricuspid valve and/or annular abscess.
  8 Check for the presence of spontaneous contrast in LA, RA, PA, and/or RV.
  9 Note presence of tricuspid valve annuloplasty ring.
  10 Note presence of pacemaker/ICD/catheter in RA and RV.
  11 Note presence of prosthetic valve in tricuspid valve position, if yes, characterize it:
    A Type: 1. bioprosthetic; 2. mechanical.
    B Rocking motion (if present suggests dehiscence).
    C Mass: 1. shape; 2. mobility; 3. size; 4. attachment site.
    D Leaflet thickness.
  12 Note presence of pericardial effusion, if present characterize its location and size.
  13 Note early diastolic collapse of RV and late diastolic early systolic collapse of RA
  (if present suspect cardiac tamponade).
  14 Check for the presence of atrial septal lipomatous hypertrophy.
  15 Note presence of atrial septal aneurysm (if present check for PFO).
  16 Note size of RA and LA.
  17 Note presence of IAS bowing to the RA or to the LA (if present suggests elevated RA or LA pressure).
  18 Note aortic valve morphology, number of cusps, sclerosis, calcification, mobility, doming, prolapse, flail.
  19 Planimetry aortic valve area if stenosis suspected.
  20 Note presence of mass, vegetation, if yes characterize it:
  1. shape; 2. mobility; 3. size; 4. attachment site.

21 Check for the presence of perivalvular abscess.
22 Note ostia of coronary vessels and their location (can help diagnose anomalous origin of the coronary ostia).
23 Note presence of prosthetic valve in aortic valve position, if present characterize the valve prosthesis:
   A Type: 1. bioprosthetic; 2. mechanical.
   B Rocking motion (if present suggests dehiscence).
   C Mass: 1. shape; 2. mobility; 3. size; 4. attachment site.
   D Leaflet thickness.
24 Note pulmonic valve morphology, mobility, thickness, calcification, coaptation, doming, flail, prolapse.
25 Note presence of mass on pulmonic valve, if yes characterize it:
   1. shape; 2. mobility; 3. size; 4. attachment site.
26 Note presence of pulmonic prosthesis if yes characterize it:
   A Type: 1. bioprosthetic; 2. mechanical.
   B Rocking motion (if present suggests dehiscence).
   C Mass: 1. shape; 2. mobility; 3. size; 4. attachment site.
   D Leaflet thickness.
27 Note spontaneous contrast in RVOT and/or main PA.
28 Measure RVOT and main PA diameters.
29 Measure right and left PA trunk diameters if visualized.
30 Check for the presence of a mass in main PA and/or proximal right and proximal left PA and if present characterize:
   1. shape; 2. mobility; 3. size; 4. attachment site.

8th: Color Doppler on parasternal 2-D short-axis view through the tricuspid, aortic and pulmonic valves
 1 Color Doppler over the tricuspid valve and RV inflow.
 2 Note presence of TR jet, if present assess
   A Eccentricity and direction.
   B Jet reaching posterior wall of RA.
   C Measure vena contracta of the TR jet.
   D Measure TR jet area and RA area, and calculate ratio.
   E Use PISA method and calculate ERO of the TR jet.
      (See the TR severity assessment in this book).
 3 Note presence of aliasing color flow during diastole over the tricuspid valve or tricuspid valve prosthesis, or annuloplasty ring (if present suspect stenosis).
 4 Note perivalvular TR in tricuspid valve prosthesis and/or presence of periannular abscess with color flow through it.
 5 Note infracristal VSD systolic jet under septal leaflet of tricuspid valve.
 6 Color Doppler over the interatrial septum: check for the presence of ASD or PFO jet.
 7 Color Doppler over the aortic valve:
   Note presence of AR jet, if present characterize:
   A Eccentricity of the jet.
   B Calculate ratio: AR jet area/aortic valve area.
   C Measure vena contracta of the AR jet.
      (See the AR severity assessment in this book.)
 8 Note presence of perivalvular abscess with color flow in it.
 9 Note presence of perivalvular AR jet in aortic valve prosthesis.

10 Color Doppler over RVOT and pulmonic valve:
   Note presence of PR jet and characterize it:
   A Eccentricity and direction.
   B Calculate width of PR jet/RVOT diameter ratio.
   C Measure vena contracta of the PR jet.
   D Length of the jet.
   (See the PR severity assessment in this book.)
11 Note systolic aliasing color Doppler in RVOT, if present suspect pulmonic stenosis or sub- or supravalvular obstruction.
12 Note systolic color flow of muscular outlet VSD in early RVOT.
13 Note systolic color flow of membranous supracristal VSD under pulmonic valve.
14 Note systolic and diastolic color Doppler flow in proximal PA in the presence of PDA.

9th: PW and CW Doppler in parasternal 2-D short-axis view through the tricuspid and pulmonic valves:

1 Check the RV diastolic inflow pattern and measure inflow velocity variation with respiration (if significant variation present suspect pathology).
2 CW Doppler through tricuspid valve:
   a Measure mean TV gradient.
   b Measure TVA by PHT method 190/PHT = TVA.
   c Measure max TR jet velocity, calculate RV/RA gradient.
   d Describe TR envelope shape (early peaking, triangular shape).
   (See the TR severity assessment in this book.)
3 CW Doppler through RVOT and pulmonic valve:
   A Note presence of PR jet.
   B Measure PAEDP gradient (absence of the late diastolic dip suggests elevated PA pressure).
   C Measure PA acceleration time and calculate mean PAD if HR allows.
   D Calculate PASP gradient and mean PV gradient.
   E Measure pressure half time of the PR jet.
   (See the PR severity assessment in this book.)

10th: 2-D parasternal short-axis view through basal level of the LV, color Doppler and M-mode scan

1 Assess LV size, function/wall motion and thickness.
2 Assess pericardial effusion presence and its size.
3 Check mitral valve leaflets structure, mobility, prolapse, calcification, coaptation, shape, presence of commissural fusion and "fish mouth" deformity suggestive of MS.
   Note MV annular calcification, abscess and presence of mass on MV, if present characterize: 1. shape; 2. mobility; 3. size; 4. attachment site.
4 With a color Doppler over the MV and identify the location of the MR jet in relation to MV scallops.
5 On M-mode tracing measure thickness of the anteroseptal and inferolateral walls during diastole and systole.

11th: 2-D parasternal short-axis view through mid LV and M-mode scan

1 Note location of papillary muscles.
2 Note segmental wall motion abnormalities and systolic thickening of the LV wall.

3 Note presence of a mass, and if present characterize:
  1. shape; 2. mobility; 3. size; 4. attachment site.
4 Note false chord presence and its attachment.
5 On M-mode scan measure LV thickness mobility, cavity size in systole and diastole.

12th: 2-D parasternal short-axis view through LV apex
1 Assess presence of LV mass, if present characterize:
  1. shape; 2. mobility; 3. size; 4. attachment site.
2 Note LV trabeculations.
3 Note segmental wall motion abnormalities and systolic thickening of the LV apex.

13th: 2-D apical 4-chambers view
1 Grossly note sizes of LV and RV, RA and LA.
2 Note LV, RV and RA, LA masses and extra structures (moderator band, false chord, and subvalvular membrane etc.), if present characterize:
  A Single vs. multiple.
  B Intramyocardial, intra- or extracavitary.
  C Mobility and size.
  D Location.
3 Note presence of spontaneous contrast in LV, RV, LA, RA.
4 Measure LA length and area.
5 Note gross LV wall thickening and segmental wall motion abnormalities if present.
6 Note pericardial thickness.
7 Note presence of pericardial effusion, if present characterize:
  Location: A. circumferential; B. loculated.
  Size: A. large; B. moderate; C. small.
8 Check for signs of cardiac tamponade:
  A Late diastolic and early systolic collapse of RA and/or LA;
  B Early diastolic collapse of the RV and/or LV.
9 Note presence of the LV true or false aneurysm, intramyocardial dissecting hematoma, if present note the location and size.
10 Note presence bioprosthetic or mechanical mitral and tricuspid valve, if present characterize:

Type of Valve	
Bioprosthetic	**Mechanical**
Carpentier-Edwards	St. Jude
Hancock	Bjork-Shiley
Other	Starr-Edwards
	Medtronic-Hall
	Other

11 Check for the stability of the prosthetic valve and absence of rocking motion.
12 Note presence of a mass on tricuspid and/or mitral prosthetic valves, if present characterize mass (zoom on it if needed):
  1. shape; 2. mobility; 3. size; 4. attachment site.
13 Check for presence of MV and/or TV annular abscess.
14 Note presence of mitral and/or tricuspid annuloplasty ring.

15 Check for the presence of IAS bowing and/or IAS aneurysm.

16 Check for the presence of IAS lipomatous hypertrophy.

17 Measure LV length and LV cavity area in systole and diastole and calculate LVEF (use additional same type of measurements done in 2-chambers view).

18 Note mitral and tricuspid valve calcification, thickening, mobility, subvalvular thickening (assign points and assess mitral valve score); Note "Hockey Stick" sign in mitral stenosis.

19 Note mitral and tricuspid valve flail leaflet(s): anterior; posterior; both leaflets.

20 Note presence of chordal and/or posterior-medial papillary muscle dysfunction/rupture.

21 Note presence of restricted motion of the MV leaflets.

22 Note presence of mass on mitral and tricuspid valves and characterize it:
A. mobility; B. size; C. attachment; D. shape.

23 Note position of tricuspid valve vs. mitral valve (check for the presence of Ebstein anomaly).

24 Note presence and assess severity of mitral and tricuspid annulus calcification.

25 Note presence of parachute mitral valve.

26 Note gross asymmetric hypertrophy of the walls.

27 Note presence of noncompaction of the ventricles.

28 Note presence of cor triatriatum.

29 Perform M-mode through basal lateral wall of the RV to measure TAPSE.

14th: Color Doppler over 4-chambers view

1 Check presence of color through the IV septum:
  A Inlet VSD upper 1/3 septum.
  B Trabecular VSD lower 2/3 septum.
  C Intramyocardial dissecting aneurysm.

2 Color through IA septum to check for the presence of right-to left or left-to-right atrial shunt.

3 Color through the apex to assess blood flow to check for the presence of: apical mass and noncompacted endocardium.

4 Color through the pseudoaneurysm to assess presence of flow.

5 Color through TV, to characterize TR jet if present:
  D. Eccentric; B. Central.
  Assess severity of the TR jet by measuring:
  A Vena contracta.
  E PISA method for ERO calculation.
  F Mosaic color flow area/RA area ratio.
   (See the TR severity assessment in this book.)

6 Note presence of periprosthetic and intravalvular TR jets.

7 Note presence of TR jet through the perforated TV leaflet.

8 Color through the annular or valvular abscess cavity if present.

9 Color through the TV, diastolic aliasing (increased velocity flow) suspect the RV inflow obstruction.

10 Color through the MV, to characterize MR jet if present:
  A. Eccentric; B. Central.
   Assess severity of the TR jet by measuring:
  A Vena contracta.
  B PISA method for ERO calculation.
  C Mosaic color flow area/LA area ratio.
   (See the MR severity assessment in this book.)

11 Color through the MV, diastolic aliasing (increased velocity flow) suspect the LV inflow obstruction;

15th: PW and CW Doppler over 4-chambers view

1 Measure MR max velocity using CW Doppler and calculate LV/LA gradient (knowing SBP of the patient LA mean pressure can be calculated, see this book).

2 Assess MV inflow Pattern with PW Doppler:
  A Impaired relaxation.
  B Pseudonormal.
  C Restrictive.
  (See diastolic function assessment in this book.)

3 Assess respiratory variation of MV inflow velocity (if significant variation present suspect pathology).

4 Measure MV maximal inflow blood velocity with CW Doppler.

5 Measure MV mean gradient if MS suspected.

6 MR jet density and shape to be noted to assess severity of MR.
  (See the MR severity assessment in this book.)

7 Measure TR max velocity using CW Doppler and calculate RV/RA gradient.

8 Assess TV inflow Pattern with PW Doppler:
  A Impaired relaxation.
  B Pseudonormal.
  C Restrictive.
  (See diastolic function assessment in this book.)

9 Assess respiratory variation of TV inflow velocity (if significant variation present suspect pathology).

10 Measure TV maximal inflow blood velocity with CW Doppler.

11 Measure TV mean gradient if TS suspected.

12 TR jet density and shape to be noted to assess severity of TR.
  (See the TR severity assessment in this book.)

13 Right upper pulmonic vein with PW Doppler to check for severity of the MR jet and help assess diastolic function of the LV.
  (See diastolic function assessment in this book.)

16th: Tissue Doppler imaging 2-D 4-chambers view

1 Tissue Doppler of the 4 segments: basal inferoseptal and basal lateral, mid inferoseptal and mid lateral; assess tissue Doppler velocities at endo- and epicardial points.
  (See assessment of LV intraventricular dyssynchrony in this book.)

2 Tissue Doppler of the basal lateral segment of the RV to assess systolic wave velocity.

17th: 2-D apical 3-chambers view

1 Zoom and measure LVOT diameter on still frame during mid to late systole if not done in parasternal long view.

2 Note presence of spontaneous contrast in RV, AO, LV, or LA.

3 Note presence of a mass in RV, AO, LV, or LA.

4 Characterize mass (zoom on it if needed):
  1. shape; 2. mobility; 3. size; 4. attachment site.

5 Check aortic wall thickness and presence of calcification.

6 Check for a proximal Aortic Dissection (presence of double lumen and intimal flap), ascending aortic aneurysm, and aortic root abscess.

7 Note presence of a mass on aortic and/or mitral valves.

8 Characterize mass (zoom on it if needed):
1. shape; 2. mobility; 3. size; 4. attachment site.

9 Note size of coronary sinus (normal < 1.5 cm).

10 Characterize LV wall segments (antero-septal: basal and mid; inferolateral: basal and mid):
1. Thickness; 2. Motion–normal vs. a. hypokinesis; b. akinesis; c. dyskinesis.

11 Note presence of an aneurysm, pseudoaneurysm and intramyocardial dissecting hematoma.

12 Note decreased amplitude of systolic aortic cusp motion due to:
A. sclerosis/stenosis; B. calcification; C. decreased stroke volume; D. HOCM; E. subvalvular stenosis.

13 Note presence of doming, prolapse and flail of aortic valve cusps.

14 Decreased amplitude of diastolic mitral valve leaflets opening due to:
A. stenosis; B. decreased stroke volume.

15 Note presence of pericardial effusion, location and qualitatively assess size:
A. anterior; B. posterior; C. circumferential.

16 Check for signs of cardiac tamponade:
A. Late diastolic and early systolic collapse of LA; B. Early diastolic collapse of the RV.

17 Check for presence of thickened and calcified pericardium.

18 Check for presence of intrapericardial mass. Characterize it:
1. shape; 2. mobility; 3. size; 4. attachment site.

19 Note calcification and its severity of mitral annulus:
1. mild; 2. moderate; 3. severe.

20 Check for the presence of mitral or aortic valve abscess.

21 Note mitral valve calcification, thickening, mobility, subvalvular thickening (assign points and assess mitral valve score). "Hockey Stick" sign in mitral stenosis.

22 Note mitral valve prolapse and/or flail: anterior; posterior; both leaflets.

23 Note presence of chordal and/or posterior-medial papillary muscle rupture.

24 Note presence of restricted motion of the MV leaflets.

25 Note presence of a posterior-medial papillary muscle dysfunction.

26 Note presence of prosthetic valve in aortic position and/or in mitral position.

Characterize valve:

Type of Valve	
Bioprosthetic	**Mechanical**
Carpentier-Edwards	St. Jude
Hancock	Bjork-Shiley
Other	Starr-Edwards
	Medtronic-Hall
	Other

27 Stability of the prosthetic valve sitting and absence of rocking.
28 Note presence of a mass on aortic and/or mitral prosthetic valves.
29 Characterize mass (zoom on it if needed):
   1. shape; 2. mobility; 3. size; 4. attachment site.
30 Check for presence of a MV annular abscess.
31 Note presence of annuloplasty ring.
32 Measure LA length and area of LA.

18th: Color Doppler over 2-D apical 3-chambers view

1 Note presence of the aortic regurgitation (AR).
2 Characterize and assess severity of the AR jet:
   a Measure width of the AR jet and calculate jet/LVOT diameter ratio.
   b Measure width of the AR jet area and calculate jet/LVOT area ratio.
   c Measure width of the vena contracta of the AR jet.
   d Comment on eccentricity and direction of the AR jet.
   (See the AR severity assessment in this book.)
3 Note presence of the mitral regurgitation (MR).
4 Characterize and assess severity of the MR jet:
   a Comment on eccentricity and direction of the MR jet.
   b Comment on length (mosaic part only) of MR jet (reaching posterior wall of LA).
   c Measure width of the vena contracta of the MR jet.
   d Measure width of the MR jet area (mosaic part only) and calculate jet/LA area ratio.
   (See the MR severity assessment in this book.)
5 Check the color flow of the blood in the dissecting septal or posterior wall if intramyocardial hematoma present.
6 Check for aliasing (high velocity) diastolic color flow of the blood through the MV inflow (suspect MV obstruction).
7 Check for aliasing (high velocity) systolic color flow of the blood through the LV outflow tract (suspect HOCM, subvalvular stenosis, AS, or intracavitary obstruction.
8 Check for presence of the color flow of the blood in proximal aortic dissection false lumen.
9 Check for presence of the perivalvular leak through aoritc and mitral valves in the presence of AV and MV prosthesis.
10 Check for presence of the aortic root and/or MV annulus communicating abscess cavity.
11 Differentiate between LV diverticulum and aneurysm based on color flow in and out of the cavity during systole and diastole (flow into the cavity during systole in the presence of aneurysm).
12 Check for the presence of MV leaflet and or aortic valve cusp perforation.

19th: PW and CW Doppler over apical 3-chambers view

1 Measure MR max velocity using CW Doppler and calculate LV/LA gradient (knowing SBP of the patient LA mean pressure can be calculated).
2 MR jet density and shape to be noted to assess severity of MR.
   (See the MR severity assessment in this book.)
3 PW Doppler through LVOT, to assess outflow tract TVI and gradient/velocity.
4 CW Doppler through LVOT and AV to assess peak and mean gradient assess the shape of envelope ("dagger").

20th: Tissue Doppler imaging 2-D apical 3-chambers view

1 Tissue Doppler of the 4 segments: basal anteroseptal and basal inferolateral, mid anteroseptal and mid infero-lateral; assess tissue Doppler velocities at endo- and epicardial points.
  (See assessment of LV intraventricular dyssynchrony in this book.)

21st: 2-D apical 2-chambers view

1 Grossly note sizes of LV and LA.

2 Note LV, LA masses and extra structures (false chord, supravalvular memrane), if present characterize:

  A Single vs. multiple.

  B Intramyocardial, intra- or extracavitary.

  C Mobility and size.

  D Location.

3 Note presence of spontaneous contrast in LV, LA.

4 Note segmental wall motion abnormalities if present (anterior and inferior walls).

5 Note pericardial thickness.

6 Note presence of pericardial effusion, if present characterize:

  Location: A. Circumferential; B. Loculated.

  Size: A. large; B. moderate; C. small.

7 Check for signs of cardiac tamponade:

  A Late diastolic and early systolic collapse of LA;

  B Early diastolic collapse of the LV.

8 Note presence of the LV true or false aneurysm, intramyocardial dissecting hematoma, if present note the location and size.

9 Note presence bioprosthetic or mechanical mitral valve, if present characterize:

Type of Valve	
Bioprosthetic	**Mechanical**
Carpentier-Edwards	St. Jude
Hancock	Bjork-Shiley
Other	Starr-Edwards
	Medtronic-Hall
	Other

10 Check for the stability of the prosthetic valve and absence of rocking motion.

11 Note presence of a mass on mitral prosthetic valve, if present characterize (zoom on it if needed):

  1. shape; 2. mobility; 3. size; 4. attachment site.

12 Check for presence of MV annular abscess.

13 Note presence of mitral annuloplasty ring.

14 Measure LV length and LV cavity area in systole and diastole and calculate LVEF (use additional same type of measurements done in 4-chambers view).

15 Note mitral and tricuspid valve calcification, thickening, mobility, subvalvular thickening (assign points and assess mitral valve score).

16 Note mitral valve flail leaflet(s): anterior; posterior; both leaflets.

17 Note presence of restricted motion of the MV leaflets.

18 Note presence of mass on mitral valve and characterize it:
   A. mobility; B. size; C. attachment site; D. shape.

19 Note presence and assess severity of mitral annulus calcification.

20 Note gross asymmetric hypertrophy of the walls.

21 Note presence of noncompaction of the ventricules.

22 Note presence of cor triatriatum.

23 Check the size of coronary sinus.

24 Check LA size, LA mass if present characterize:
   A. mobility; B. size; C. attachment; D. shape.

22nd: Color Doppler over 2-D apical 2-chambers view

1 Note presence of the mitral regurgitation (MR).

2 Characterize the MR jet:
   A Comment on eccentricity and direction of the MR jet.
   B Comment on length (mosaic part only) of MR jet (reaching posterior wall of LA).

3 Check the color Doppler flow of the blood in the dissecting anterior or inferior wall if intramyocardial hematoma present.

4 Check the color Doppler flow of the blood in the anterior or inferior wall if pseudoaneurysm present.

5 Check for aliasing (high velocity) diastolic color Doppler flow of the blood through the MV inflow (suspect MV obstruction).

6 Check for presence of the perivalvular leak through Mitral valve in the presence of MV prosthesis.

7 Check for presence of the MV annulus communicating abscess cavity.

8 Differentiate between LV diverticulum and aneurysm based on color Doppler flow in and out of the cavity during systole and diastole (flow into the cavity during systole in the presence of aneurysm).

9 Check for the presence of MV leaflet and or aortic valve cusp perforation.

23rd: Tissue Doppler imaging over 2-D apical 2-chambers view

1 Tissue Doppler of the 4 segments: basal anterior and basal inferior, mid anterior and mid inferior; assess tissue Doppler velocities at endo- and epicardial points.
   (See assessment of LV intraventricular dyssynchrony in this book.)

24th: 2-D apical 5-chambers view

1 Note LV, RV and RA, LA masses and extra structures (moderator band, false chord, supra- and subvalvular membrane etc.), if present characterize:
   A Single vs. multiple.
   B Intramyocardial, intra- or extracavitary.
   C Mobility and size.
   D Location.

2 Note presence of spontaneous contrast in LV, RV, LA, RA.

3 Note pericardial thickness.

4 Note presence of pericardial effusion, if present characterize:
   Location: A. circumferential; B. loculated.
   Size: A. large; B. moderate; C. small.

5 Note presence bioprosthetic or mechanical mitral and aortic valve, if present characterize:

Type of Valve	
Bioprosthetic	**Mechanical**
Carpentier-Edwards	St. Jude
Hancock	Bjork-Shiley
Other	Starr-Edwards
	Medtronic-Hall
	Other

6 Check for the stability of the prosthetic valve and absence of rocking motion.
7 Note presence of a mass on aortic and/or mitral prosthetic valves, if present characterize mass (zoom on it if needed):
   1. shape; 2. mobility; 3. size; 4. attachment site.
8 Check for presence of annular abscess.
9 Note presence of mitral annuloplasty ring.
10 Note mitral and aortic valve calcification, thickening, and mobility.
11 Note mitral and aortic valve flail leaflet(s).
12 Note presence of restricted motion of the MV leaflets.
13 Note presence of mass on mitral and aortic valves and characterize it:
   A. mobility; B. size; C. attachment; D. shape.
14 Note presence and assess severity of mitral annulus calcification.

25th: Color Doppler over 2-D apical 5-chambers view
1 Note presence of the aortic regurgitation (AR).
2 Characterize and assess severity of the AR jet:
3 Measure width of the AR jet and calculate jet/LVOT diameter ratio.
4 Measure width of the AR jet area and calculate jet/LVOT area ratio.
   a Measure width of the vena contracta of the AR jet.
   b Comment on eccentricity and direction of the AR jet.
      (See the AR severity assessment in this book.)
5 Note presence of the mitral regurgitation (MR).
6 Characterize the MR jet.
7 Comment on eccentricity and direction of the MR jet.
8 Comment on length (mosaic part only) of MR jet (reaching posterior wall of LA).
9 Check for aliasing (high velocity) diastolic color flow of the blood through the MV inflow (suspect MV obstruction).
10 Check for aliasing (high velocity) systolic color Doppler flow of the blood through the LV outflow tract (suspect HOCM, subvalvular stenosis) or intracavitary obstruction.
11 Check for presence of ventricular septal defect (VSD) color jet in systole from LV to RV.
12 Check for presence of the color Doppler flow of the blood in proximal aortic dissection false lumen.
13 Check for presence of the perivalvular leak through aortic and mitral valves in the presence of AV and/or MV prosthesis.

14 Check for presence of the aortic root and/or MV annulus communicating abscess cavity.
15 Check for the presence of MV leaflet and or aortic valve cusp perforation;

26th: PW and CW Doppler over 2-D apical 5-chambers view

1 Measure MR max velocity using CW Doppler and calculate LV/LA gradient (knowing SBP of the patient, LA mean pressure can be calculated, see this book).
2 MR jet density and shape to be noted to assess severity of MR
   (See the MR severity assessment in this book.)
3 PW Doppler through LVOT, to assess outflow tract TVI and gradient/velocity.
4 CW Doppler through LVOT and AV to assess peak and mean gradient and assess the shape of envelope ("dagger").

27th: 2-D subcostal view (long-axis view)

1 Grossly note sizes of LV and RV, RA and LA.
2 Note LV, RV and RA, LA masses and extra structures (moderator band, false chord, supra- and subvalvular membrane etc.), if present characterize:
   b Single vs. multiple.
   c Intramyocardial, intra-or extracavitary.
   d Mobility and size.
   e Location.
3 Note presence of spontaneous contrast in LV, RV, LA, RA.
4 Note pericardial thickness.
5 Note presence of pericardial effusion, if present characterize:
   Location: A. circumferential; B. loculated.
   Size: A. large; B. moderate; C. small.
6 Check for signs of cardiac tamponade:
   A Late diastolic and early systolic collapse of RA and/or LA;
   B Early diastolic collapse of the RV and/or LV.
7 Note presence of the LV true or false aneurysm, intramyocardial dissecting hematoma, if present note the location and size.
8 Note presence of bioprosthetic or mechanical mitral and tricuspid valve, if present characterize:

Type of Valve	
Bioprosthetic	**Mechanical**
Carpentier-Edwards	St. Jude
Hancock	Bjork-Shiley
Other	Starr-Edwards
	Medtronic-Hall
	Other

9 Check for the stability of the prosthetic valve sitting and absence of rocking.
10 Note presence of a mass on tricuspid and/or mitral prosthetic Valves, if present characterize mass (zoom on it if needed):
   1. shape; 2. mobility; 3. size; 4. attachment site.
11 Check for presence of MV and/or TV annular abscess.

12 Note presence of mitral and/or tricuspid annuloplasty ring.

13 Check for the presence of IAS bowing and/or IAS aneurysm.

14 Check for the presence of IAS lipomatous hypertrophy.

15 Note mitral and tricuspid valve calcification, thickening, mobility.

16 Note mitral and tricuspid valve flail leaflet(s): anterior; posterior; both leaflets.

17 Note presence of restricted motion of the MV leaflets.

18 Note presence of mass on mitral and tricuspid valves and characterize it:
A. mobility; B. size; C. attachment; D. shape.

19 Note position of tricuspid valve vs. mitral valve (check for the presence of Ebstein anomaly).

20 Note presence and assess severity of mitral and tricuspid annulus calcification.

21 Note gross asymmetric hypertrophy of the walls.

22 Note presence of noncompaction of the ventricles.

23 Note presence of cor triatriatum.

24 Contrast injection to assess presence and severity of PFO, ASD.

25 Measure size and effect of inspiration on diameter of IVC to assess the RA pressure (see this book).

26 Note presence of pacemaker/ICD/catheter in RA and RV.

28th: Subcostal 2-D short-axis view through the aortic valve

1 Comment on tricuspid valve leaflets:
A. structure; B. mobility; C. thickness, D. calcification; E. coaptation; F. flail and prolapse.

2 Note presence of RV, RA and/or LA mass.

3 Characterize the mass if present:
1. shape; 2. mobility; 3. size; 4. attachment site.

4 Note presence of Eustachian valve and Chiari network.

5 Note presence of tricuspid valve mass and characterize it if present:
1. shape; 2. mobility; 3. size; 4. attachment site.

6 Check for the presence of tricuspid valve and/or annular abscess.

7 Check for the presence of spontaneous contrast in LA, RA, PA, and/or RV.

8 Note presence of tricuspid valve annuloplasty ring.

9 Note presence of pacemaker/ICD/catheter in RA and RV.

10 Note presence of prosthetic valve in tricuspid valve position, if yes, characterize it:
A Type: 1. bioprosthetic; 2. mechanical.
B Rocking motion (if present suggests dehiscence).
C Mass: 1. shape; 2. mobility; 3. size; 4. attachment site.
D Leaflet thickness.

11 Note presence of pericardial effusion, if present characterize its location and size.

12 Note early diastolic collapse of RV and late diastolic early systolic collapse of RA (if present suspect cardiac tamponade).

13 Check for the presence of atrial septal lipomatous hypertrophy.

14 Note presence of atrial septal aneurysm (if present check for PFO).

15 Note presence of IAS bowing to the RA or to the LA (if present suggests elevated RA or LA pressure).

16 Note aortic vale morphology, number of cusps, sclerosis, calcification, mobility, prolapse, flail.

17 Planimetry aortic valve area if stenosis suspected.

18 Note presence of mass, vegetation, if yes characterize it:
1. shape; 2. mobility; 3. size; 4. attachment site.

19 Check for the presence of perivalvular abscess.
20 Note ostia of coronary vessels and their location (can help diagnose anomalous origin of the coronary ostia).
21 Note presence of prosthetic valve in aortic valve position, if present characterize the valve prosthesis:
   A Type: 1. bioprosthetic; 2. mechanical.
   B Rocking motion (if present suggests dehiscence).
   C Mass: 1. shape; 2. mobility; 3. size; 4. attachment site.
   D Leaflet thickness.
22 Note pulmonic valve morphology, mobility, thickness, calcification, coaptation, doming, flail, prolapse.
23 Note presence of mass on pulmonic valve, if yes characterize it:
   1. shape; 2. mobility; 3. size; 4. attachment site.
24 Note presence of pulmonic prosthesis if yes characterize it:
   A Type: 1. bioprosthetic; 2. mechanical.
   B Rocking motion (if present suggests dehiscence).
   C Mass: 1. shape; 2. mobility; 3. size; 4. attachment site.
   D Leaflet thickness.
25 Note spontaneous contrast in RVOT and/or main PA.
26 Measure RVOT and main PA diameters.
27 Measure right and left PA trunk diameters if visualized.
28 Check for the presence of a mass in main PA and/or proximal right and proximal left PA, if present characterize:
   1. shape; 2. mobility; 3. size; 4. attachment site.

29th: Subcostal 2-D short axis view through basal level of the LV, color Doppler scan

1 Assess LV size, function/wall motion and thickness.
2 Assess pericardial effusion presence and its size.
3 Check mitral valve leaflets structure, mobility, prolapse, calcification, coaptation, shape, presence of commissural fusion and "fish mouth" deformity suggestive of MS presence.
   Note MV annular calcification and presence mass on MV, if present characterize:
   1. shape; 2. mobility; 3. size; 4. attachment site.
4 With a color Doppler over the MV identify the location of the MR jet in relation to MV scallops.

30th: 2-D Subcostal short-axis view through mid LV and M-mode scan

1 Note segmental wall motion abnormalities if present and systolic thickening of the LV wall.
2 Note presence of a mass, and if present characterize:
   1. shape; 2. mobility; 3. size; 4. attachment site.
3 Note false chord presence and its attachment.

31st: 2-D Subcostal short axis view through LV apex

1 Assess presence of LV mass, if present characterize.
   1. shape; 2. mobility; 3. size; 4. attachment site.
2 Note LV trabeculations.
3 Note segmental wall motion abnormalities if present and systolic thickening of the LV apex.

32nd: Subcostal 2-D and PW Doppler view

1 Measure the diameter of IVC and effect of inspiration on it, to assess RAP.
   (See estimation of RA pressure in this book.)

2 PW Doppler of hepatic veins and effect of inspiration/expiration on the amplitude of Doppler waves.

33rd: Suprasternal 2-D long, color and PW/CW Doppler view

1 Identify presence of ascending or descending aortic dissection:
   1. false lumen; 2. intimal flap.

2 Check color Doppler flow in ascending and descending aorta.

3 Check PW Doppler flow in descending aorta, if holodiastolic flow documented suspect presence of severe AR.

4 Check CW Doppler flow in ascending aorta if high velocity jet documented suspect obstruction (valvular stenosis, sub- or supravalvular stenosis, dynamic LVOT or intracavitary obstruction).

5 Check CW Doppler flow in descending aorta if velocity is increased obstruction suspected (aortic coarctation).